Positude Paramedic

4 Strategies, 5 Skills, and 100 Experiences to Becoming a Positude Paramedic

Walter Dusseldorp

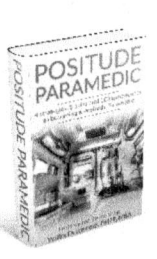

Dusseldorp & Associates, Inc.
107 Strawtown Road
New City, NY 10956
(646) 208–5217
www.positudeleadership.com

Copyright © 2017 Walter Dusseldorp

ISBN-13: 978-1539709084
ISBN-10: 1539709086

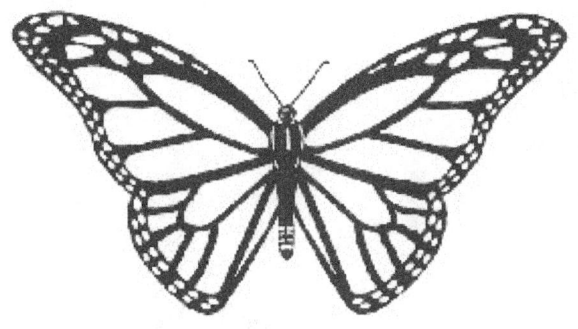

Dedicated to a sweet soul taken from us all too soon:

Larisa Karassik

#28

www.larisastrong.org

Don't Drink and Drive!

Contents

- Fire Medic
- Community Paramedic
- Long-Term Goals Postparamedicine

Part II: Five Skills

5. Skill 1: Partnerships
   - Communication Skills
   - Building Vital Partnerships
   - Critical Feedback
   - Stress Debriefing

6. Skill 2: Situational Awareness
   - Safety First
   - Being Aware of Your Surroundings
   - Emergency Response
   - Incident Command
   - Emergency Management

7. Skill 3: Patient Assessment
   - Introduction
   - Creating a Safe Environment
   - Asking the Right Questions
   - Head-to-Toe Exam
   - Nonverbal Communication
   - Each Assessment Tells a Story

8. Skill 4: Patient Care
   a. Medical Emergencies
   b. Traumatic Emergencies

9. Skill 5: Medication Management
   - Medication Reconciliation
   - Drug Calculations
   - Medication Resource Management

Part III: Special Contributors

10. Medical Direction and EMS
    - Jeffrey Rabrich, DO, FACEP, EMT-P

11. Medical Legal Consideration: So Help Me God?
    - Joel Hirshfield, Esq., EMTP

12. From EMT to MD
    - Sean Kivlehan, MD

13. So You Want to Be a Wilderness Paramedic
    - Frank DiGianni, NREMTP

14. A Woman's Perspective
    - Lieutenant Bernadette Frae, BS, EMT-Paramedic

15. Responding to a Terrorism-Related Incident: All-Hazards Approach All the Time
    - Steven Kanarian, FDNY EMS EMT-Paramedic

16. Family Tragedy "Survivor Story"
    - The Riello Family

Part IV: One Hundred Experiences

Conclusion

Special Recognition

Just to make sure that I don't leave anybody out, I'm sincerely grateful for *all* my partners over the years. I learned from each of you, and collectively you all have made me a better person, leader, and paramedic.

Over the past twenty-six years, some of you made special contributions worth special recognition and mention:

Boomer Bojo—My first real partner in EMS: "Brothers Forever."

Shawn Kauffman—My first EMS boss. Nobody documents better than you!

HVCC Dan Olsen, Richard Beebe, and Greg Chapman—Best paramedic CICs.

Dick Jones—For sending me on my first ALS (advanced life support) job five minutes after you hired me.

Edward Horton—For believing in me and developing me as a young manager.

Mike Murphy—For bringing me to Rockland Paramedics in 1993.

Nick Veltri—For being my brother in my early formative years.

Vincent Romano—For taking the time to teach me "Investing 101."

Bernadette Frae—For being my "work" wife for the past fifteen years.

Joel Hirshfield—For being my big brother and partner in crime.

Dr. Markowitz—For allowing me to get away with it.

Dr. Michael S. Lippe—For sharing and elevating EMS standards of care.

Dr. Erik Larsen—For hiring me onto the flight team..."Best Job Ever."

Chrissie Murphy—For being the best, funniest, and coolest flight nurse.

Frank DiGianni—For being my best man and being a great older brother.

Bill Palmer, Bill Pope, David Lichtbach, and Charlie Robinson—For keeping us safe while flying around the Hudson Valley. Each of you is awesome in your own right.

Preface

The Future of Paramedicine

I wished upon a star that I had the ability to stare into a glass ball and see the future of paramedicine. Nope, that didn't work. Let's try it the traditional way then, through market analysis, discussion, and literature review. I don't want to bore you with complex studies and statistics, but let me try to summarize and pontificate on where I think paramedicine is heading over the next five years.

To stave off an argument, I'm going to assume that our nursing union friends are not going to obstruct progress in the field of paramedicine and the likely excursion into community paramedics.

For starters, I believe that the paramedic profession is finally becoming a recognized career path with multiple options to choose from, including transport, critical care, 911, and flight medicine. However, we have a long way to go to make it a career path that can sustain an average-size family while only working forty hours per week. Salary disparity continues to make it a major struggle in paramedicine to retain the finest and brightest minds. Because of the constant brain drain, many agencies find themselves struggling to retain and train the next generation.

More importantly, we need to elevate our profession by mandating a paramedic bachelor degree. Preferably, paramedics should become a recognized third service mandated by all municipalities to maintain a high standard of care for its citizens. Lastly, we need to set new standards for pay parity across the country. A combination of these efforts will allow our profession to become a career.

To be considered a career path, we need to add several layers to allow paramedics to work at different intensity levels depending on age, form, and desired function. What do we need to do to establish a base for our future? We need to develop programs around community paramedicine, behavioral health, and occupational health medicine. Each of these programs can be delivered at a much lower cost and be truly preventative in nature.

Since I will discuss the more traditional service lines for paramedics in much greater detail later, I'm going to spend a paragraph here on each of the three new service lines identified above.

Community paramedicine is not a new concept; however, it is yet to be fully embraced or even funded by the Centers of Medicare and Medicaid Services. Some of the most rural areas of the United States have advanced paramedics covering these small communities to provide basic health checkups, update vaccinations, and respond to minor medical emergencies. The next level of community paramedicine will be attained only after insurance companies realize that it's less expensive to care for their patients outside the four walls of a hospital. This is especially true in remote corners of the country and in high-density neighborhoods where patients tend to depend on their local emergency rooms for primary care.

Supported by technologies such as advanced portable diagnostics and telemedicine, community paramedics can fill a gap that currently exists in most communities. High-risk frequent users of emergency services respond well to intermittent supportive care at their homes given by visiting nurse services and ability-activated community paramedics prior to choosing to go to the hospital. Paramedics are the perfect vehicles for urgent care in the home, providing short interactions at a relatively low cost. It is also a great opportunity for the transitioning paramedic—going from an intense 911-response unit to a preventative setting is less stressful on the aging body and mind.

I have worked in New York City for the past five years, and it is more apparent to me than ever that many of our patients have a strong behavioral component along with their other chronic diseases. It's a combination that is a predictor of poor control over their hypertension, diabetes, asthma, and kidney disease, not to mention obesity, which is often the predictor of aforesaid chronic diseases.

Today, we treat these diseases in our primary practices and often learn only after the fact that patient went to the emergency room for treatment. Needless to say, this comes at a significant cost to society. We need to make a transformative change to address this massive burden on our Medicare and Medicaid budgets.

In the not-too-distant future, a specialty line of paramedics should be developed that will position paramedics to manage chronic diseases plus the patients' associated mental illness. This treatment should preferably be provided in the patients' natural environment such as their homes or community centers. These especially trained paramedics will have the ability to de-escalate acute onset psychosis or mitigate the patients' underlying mental illness condition without the need to transport them to the nearest CPEP unit and/or in-patient admission.

Last but not least, the occupational health paramedic could become the next revenue opportunity for existing paramedic services or a cost-reduction opportunity for managed-care providers. This type of paramedic would concentrate on preventative care, nutrition, and weight and exercise management in the workplace. Your next employer might want to hire an occupational health paramedic to reduce variable overhead expenses such as the cost of health-care insurance. Employers currently offer reduced-cost gym membership plans to entice employees to adopt a healthier lifestyle. The premise is right; however, the approach falls short of guaranteeing success due to the fact that most employees lack the behavioral capacity to follow through on regular exercise. This is especially true for those who could benefit from it most.

This is when the occupational paramedic comes to the rescue. Regardless of if the paramedic is a hired gun or part of the organization, this role is vital to providing consistent access to health monitoring, exercise, and even rehabilitation.

As a society, we are reactive in our responses and don't invest enough time, money, or effort in prevention, especially in the formative years of our future patients. Paramedics are uniquely positioned to take on the role as early interventionists and prescreeners before emergency medical services (EMS) is activated.

An ounce of prevention is worth its weight in gold. Together we can do more!

Introduction

How I Came to *Love* the Art of Medicine

It all started on the day I was born. Six weeks early and weighing only four pounds, four ounces, I fit into my father's large hands. Being in the hospital for the first few weeks of my life must have had a lasting impression on me.

In my adolescent years, I had too many encounters with the medical system—according to my mom, that is. Since I only knew one speed (fast), I frequently ended up with injuries that required visits to the doctor's office or, on some occasions, the emergency room. After a few fractures, sprains, and lacerations, I was well acquainted with Dr. Ubachs, our hometown doctor, one of the old-fashioned kinds who came to your house when you were too sick to come to his practice.

We hit it off on day one. In my recollection, he wanted me to take over his medical practice when he was ready to retire (not sure how many other kids he promised this to as well). Regardless, it made a lasting impression on me, and even to this day, I think of him or mention him on regular basis.

Life took a few twists and turns along the way, which distracted me from pursuing my first love and aspiration to be just like Dr. Ubachs.

As a teenager, I did get involved with EHBO (the Dutch version of the American Red Cross's first-aid training) and met a lovely and kind woman by the name of Maria. She provided great mentorship and guided me through some turbulent waters. I truly enjoyed studying and applying what we learned. Not unlike many others, I chased every ambulance that came through town to get a glimpse of the professionals at work. When the opportunity arose, I jumped into action to assist however I could, whether it was applying a Band-Aid, taking care of sick folks at parties, or occasionally helping an injured player on the field.

My fate was sealed the day I was returning from school in the afternoon and came upon a bicyclist who had been struck by a car going at a high rate of speed. This elderly man—I still remember it like it was yesterday—was bleeding profusely from his head. He muttered some sounds—I'm not sure if they were even actual words. I placed my ungloved hands under his head to get it off the pavement, and I felt my fingers slip into his skull. Not sure what to do, I pulled back and held his head stable until professional help arrived. Right there and then, I knew that I wanted to be a paramedic. I officially caught the bug and have yet to find an antidote that will cure me and pull me away from it.

If you asked ten of your closest friends in EMS or emergency medicine about why they got into the field, you would likely hear similar stories or about their exposure to early childhood diseases that led them to pursue a career in medicine.

I have now been involved with emergency services for nearly thirty years and don't have a single regret. It's been a hard, exciting life that has taken its toll on my body and mind. I can truly reflect back on the decades and find far more good than bad. I have lots of reasons to be very proud, and I believe that I have made a difference a few times along the way.

Transition: Getting into the Right Mind-Set

Before we transition to the core of *Positude Paramedic*, I just want to take a few minutes to outline what you should expect in the book. This will ensure that you have a better reading experience. This handbook is meant to provide guidance to aspiring paramedics as well as show ways for current paramedics and technicians to improve the way they deliver care to their patients. The one hundred deep personal-experience stories are supposed to provide a glimpse into what it is actually like to be a paramedic and to provide guidance on how to be a better paramedic.

If you apply the book's four strategies and five skills appropriately, you are more likely to make the right choices and become a paramedic with a great attitude or *positude.*

There are embedded "tool kits" in the text for you to use to continue to explore career-path options, such as identifying colleges that offer a paramedic program. These tool kits will guide you through some questions that will help you make an informed decision. We will have similar exercises for career planning, building lasting partnerships, and guiding you on how to get the best results.

We strive to establish the four foundational principles for long-term success:

1. Unwavering mutual respect for each other
2. Common bond—Why we do it
3. Common understanding—When we do it
4. Maintaining a teachable attitude

Most importantly, have fun, be mindful of your mindfulness, feel inspired, and be inspiring.

Part I: Four Strategies

1

Strategy 1: Developing Career Options

Getting to Know Yourself First

For argument's sake, we will assume that you are at the point in your life when you are exploring career options but that you have no clue where to start. There are so many options to choose from. Aligning your passion with a career opportunity should be your primary driver at this point in time.

Before you select a career path, you need to learn more about yourself: what gets you excited, what grabs your interest, what types of jobs you have been exposed to, or even better, what you wonder about but have never had the opportunity to explore.

Professional satisfaction should be your aim, not money alone. I have many friends who go to work each day and are making lots of money but hate what they do. Life is too short not to pursue your dreams or pursue a career path that will meet your intrinsic values and allow you to leave home each day with a big, bright smile on your face. I'm the luckiest guy on this earth—I truly *love* what I do!

Getting started could be a bit overwhelming, and it should not be a decision you make on the fly. Deep thought and hard work should deliver results that will bring professional happiness for life. Being a *positude* anything in life requires you to be highly enthusiastic and passionate about your work.

So let's do some hard work and complete Tool Kit #1 to help you find out what you are truly passionate about.

Since you are reading this book, I'm going to use medicine as a pathway example.

Tool Kit #1

Finding the *RIGHT* career for me!

Sector	Category	Career	Passion
Medicine	EMT	BLS Ambulance	
	Paramedic	Transport 911 Critical care Flight	
	Nurse	Emergency Med-surg Critical care Behavior	
	Physician Assistant	General Surgical Private	
	Doctor	Medicine Surgical Behavioral OB-GYN Emergency	
	Technician	Radiology Respiratory Nursing	

Depending on your school grades, be very realistic in your approach to finding the right opportunity to explore. Each requires independent research on your part, and if possible, explore options to complete a ride-along, internship, or volunteer assignment or to be able to shadow or interview folks who are currently in these positions.

Don't rush through this section: You are going to make a choice for life. Since we only get to live one life, make the right choice for yourself.

This is an introspective exercise about yourself; however, it would not be complete if you fail to bring others into the loop.

Completing a 360-Degree Assessment

To get to know yourself, you need to learn from those around you. A 360-degree assessment means literally asking folks all around you for their opinion and allowing them to share valuable lifetime experiences that you can learn from. Even more importantly, folks who know you best can help you recognize your own strengths and weaknesses. This is not an easy exercise, especially for young folks in their late teens or early twenties when their emotional maturity is not at a level where critical feedback is appreciated or valued.

Part of getting to know yourself is understanding what you are not good at. However, it is essential from a learning perspective and also affects your abilities to make the right choices along the way.

To make the most out of this exercise, include people whom you don't necessarily like or agree with. After your first tool-kit exercise, you found an area of interest, such as medicine; however, perhaps you are not quite sure if you have what it takes to become a doctor, nurse, or paramedic.

Instead of going forward without exploring others' opinions about yourself that might assist you in your decision-making process, let's get started by identifying whom you should interview from a 360-degree perspective. Let's assume that you are finishing high school or some college but remain undecided on your major. Use this example as your starting point for interviewees:

1. Parents
2. Siblings
3. Aunts/uncles
4. Best friends
5. Long-time neighbors
6. Early childhood teacher
7. High-school teacher
8. Sporting coach
9. Guidance counselor or mentor
10. Other

It may seem like a lot of work. However, fifteen minutes with each person is invaluable when you are going to make a decision for a lifetime. Trying to get it right the first time around will prevent unnecessary cost and mental anguish. If nothing else, your relationship with each will be elevated to another level of respect, and you will receive an awesome building block to strengthen your own emotional maturity.

Invest in yourself wisely and conduct a full 360-degree assessment using Tool Kit #2, outlined on the next page.

Tool Kit #2

SWOT Analysis

Example 360-degree assessment interview: Father

Make a thirty-minute appointment a week in advance and provide a short description for the intended meeting. This will allow the interviewee to be thoughtful and ready at time of your meeting.

Category	Findings	Summary
Strengths	Determined	
	Driven	
	Reserved	
	Analytic	
	Kind to others	
Weaknesses	Public speaking	
	Short attention span	
	Shy	
	Doesn't like blood	
Opportunities	Public speaking	
	Finance	
	Health care	
	Management	
	Accounting	
	Music	
Threats	Competitive	
	Limited jobs	
	Low pay	

After you have completed all of your 360 assessments, merge them together and look for commonalities. Use this to strengthen your weaknesses, explore your opportunities, and determine which workforce category speaks most to your strengths. Go back to Tool Kit #1 and repeat the exercise to see if you have changed your mind or solidified what you already know about yourself.

Making a Commitment

This is one of the most important decisions you will ever make besides marrying the right person and buying your first house.

If you are graduating high school and are not sure of your direction even after completing Tool Kits #1 and #2, commit to college by taking general coursework with a concentration in the areas that interest you. Don't wait too long before making a commitment to your future. If possible, find a volunteer intern position for weekends, holidays, and between semesters. This will allow you to get a glimpse "under the hood," which could be a worthy investment in yourself.

If you have decided and are ready to commit, *focus* will need to become your next best friend going forward. Although I encourage you to live a full life with lots of fun and exploration, focus is a necessity if you are to accomplish your goals.

Before you commit, perform one last fact assessment to ensure your goal meets the following requirements:

Specific

Measureable

Attainable

Realistic

Timely

Meeting your SMART goals will increase your success rate and prevent you from overreaching, if done correctly.

Creating an Action Plan

Up to this point in time, it's been all talk and little action or at least no action planning. Assuming that you have come to some conclusion about your future (now or in the future), it will take focus and a great plan in order to reach success.

If you don't plan well in advance and take lots of variables into consideration, you will probably win a battle or two but likely will lose the war. In other words, if you don't connect the dots as you proceed through your education, you will likely not end up where you wanted to go originally. Now, to be fair, as life progresses, you will gain new beliefs and experiences that could potentially alter your original course.

The main lesson to be learned in creating an action plan is the fact that you need to have your desired results in mind. Your personal experiences will create beliefs that lead you to take action that delivers certain results. If you want to change the results, you will need to change your actions.

Life is a series of projects that require careful planning and execution. At times, you can work on multiple facets at the same time, while at other times one will need to be done before the next. While building a house, you need to have a strong foundation before you can build the house on top of it. However, to be efficient, the plumber should lay out water, sewer, and gas lines before the concrete is poured. It's no different in your educational goals. You will have to take certain prerequisites before taking higher-level coursework. If you are in a highly competitive program with limited room in each course offering, you will need to stay on top of release dates to be first in line.

For additional resources, Google the search term "Gantt chart" to see examples of project-planning tools. There are a lot of choices available online, or you can simply create one of your own.

Since this handbook is for paramedics, from this point forward I'm going to assume that you are an emergency medical technician (EMT) looking for career advancement.

If you are not yet an EMT, I highly recommend that you contact your local office of emergency management. Inquire about the best ways to become an EMT and ways you can contribute now. There are too many variables to describe in this chapter; however, in New York State most volunteer ambulance services will pay for you to attend an EMT course and will require you to volunteer about twelve hours per week.

You *must* be an EMT before you can become a paramedic. Even if they didn't mandate this, I highly recommend you get your feet wet while volunteering or working for your local paid EMS provider. This will allow you to gain valuable experience and to get a really good look up close before you make your final commitment to becoming a paramedic.

If you are in the transition year between finishing your bachelor of science degree and beginning medical school, taking a paramedic course is well worth your time and the investment. You will definitely have a leg up on all the others who came straight from their undergraduate degree without any exposure to emergency service.

Tool Kit #3

Google "Gantt Chart"

Lay out an educational plan that will deliver your desired result.

Think of building a house. You have to level the ground and lay out your plumbing before pouring the foundation. Doing it out of sequence will cause significantly more work or expenses or even failure of the project.

A Gantt chart is a powerful visual tool that serves to keep you organized and at the same time assist you with communicating your project status.

Gantt Chart - Project Schedule

Task Name	ID	January																		
		1	2	3	4	5	6	7	8	9	10	11	12	13	14	15	16	17	18	19
Do Initial Design	1																			
Price Design	2																			
Order Materials	3																			

2

Strategy 2: Selecting the Right Program

Ranking of Programs

Just because it advertises itself as a paramedic program doesn't necessarily make it a great program. Don't just assume that it is the right program for you just because it is nearest to where you live or work.

It's not unlike shopping for your next new car. You need to know what you want to get out of it and gauge the options against your standards.

I would suggest contacting your state health department's emergency services division and request a listing of all approved paramedic programs. If you live near state borders, you might have to reach out to each state's respective office to make an informed decision.

Before meeting with any of the program directors, create a list based on your needs. For example, you may need the program to be less than one hundred miles from home, have a graduation rate higher than 90 percent, have a program history of ten years or longer, have an accredited or established AS or BS program, and so on.

Based on your own parameters, generate a list of your top three programs. Contact each program director and request a face-to-face meeting to discuss his or her respective paramedic programs.

Make sure that you are prepared for this meeting as it will be a bilateral discussion. You are interested in learning about the program from someone who is its primary salesperson. By the same token, the program director gets a glimpse of you as a potential paramedic student.

Interviewing with the Program Director

You have applied to several programs, and now it's time for you be interviewed by the program director. It will be up to the director whether or not to accept you into the program. If you have done your homework well, you applied to highly competitive programs where there will be more applicants than positions available.

It's show time; all the effort in getting ready to select the right program is now going to pay off. It's time to be focused in your responses and show that you have great interpersonal skills as well as have the ability to listen intently and provide crisp answers to basic questions.

You should anticipate and practice answering the top five most common questions. Prepare short power statements that show that you have carefully thought out your responses (but be careful that you say them without sounding too robotic).

Let's pick five common questions. However, feel free to expand upon these.

1. Why do you want to be a paramedic?
2. What have you done to prepare to join our program?
3. What are your core strengths and weaknesses?
4. What are your study habits?
5. How well do you work under stress?

Your answers should be about thirty to forty-five seconds in length with a beginning, a middle, and a power end.

I also recommend that you prepare a personal value statement. Mine is as follows:

> *I'm a leader who aspires to lead with great humility in a servant-like, collaborative manner. Patient safety and quality of care are the most important to me.*

After all your interviews, summarize your experiences and learn from each one. Always believe that you can create opportunities from failure. Your personal experiences with each program director will be an important factor in your final selection process.

Making Your Final Selection

It's time to go back to Tool Kit #2's SWOT analysis. Now, use your findings to evaluate what strengths, weaknesses, and opportunities each program offers. You should pay special attention to the threats in this case, such as low graduation rates, frequent staff turnover, financially poor conditions, weak affiliation with accredited colleges, and so on.

Once you have done your homework and discussed it with your mentor, you are ready to commit and apply to your program of choice.

3

Strategy 3: Becoming a Paramedic

Studying with Great Focus

Trust me when I say that if you don't get organized right from day one, you will feel overwhelmed with information and the tasks at hand.

Depending on what type of paramedic program you have selected, your classes will be distributed over either two or four semesters. This on its own is not that difficult since the rest of the student body is experiencing the same thing.

What is different from most other programs is your requirement to complete ride-along time with paramedics plus many hours of rotations through different specialties in the hospital.

The best way to approach your next one to two years is through great focus. You have to adopt a strategy of "nothing else matters" if you want to be the best. It's perfectly fine to take focused time off from studying or even taking a short break for vacation to recharge. However, it is simply a bad idea to treat completing a paramedic program as second priority to partying.

Your personal value statement, which was developed in the previous chapter, is your guiding light to become a great paramedic and a *Positude* Paramedic.

Great focus, or being in the moment, will especially allow you to get the best experiences during your rotations. You will only get out of it what you put into it. Every program has someone who thinks the program and requirements are just a cakewalk only to fail out at some point in time. Don't let that be you.

Adopt a positive attitude (*positude*) as you move forward from this point on. This allows you to be respectful, mindful, and teachable, which are key ingredients to working and studying with great focus.

Now that your mind-set is *positude*, working with great focus requires one more consideration. Work on only one to two projects at any given time. Working on three to five projects simultaneously minimizes success, and working on more than five leads to failure.

Your organizational skills will need to be on steroids to stay ahead of the game. Using a project-management tool such as a Gantt chart will allow you to schedule your time and effort on focused projects (subjects/topics) to ensure a higher degree of success in each one.

Why am I making a big deal about focus? Simply, I am talking about the patient care that you will eventually be delivering to my friends, family, and neighbors. I want you to be the very best paramedic—if you learned to focus while studying, in times of emergency you can focus on the subject at hand.

After all is said and done, focus on patient safety and quality delivery of care. That is what it is all about.

Listening versus Writing Notes

With the hope that the last few pages have sunk in and you can now see why focus is such an important factor to your success, let's delve into an area of great discussion and variability between students.

At this point in your career or student life, all of you have been in lecture halls large or small to listen to an instructor or professor. The question is: Did you really listen or just hear what was said? Another question is: Did you take copious notes while they were lecturing or just a few words?

Only you can answer that question honestly for yourself. However, I can make some assumptions based on research and deep personal experiences.

The vast majority of you hears but doesn't really listen to all that is said due to lack of focus, disinterest in the topic, or a short attention span. There's always someone in the class who is an awesome notetaker who has the ability to listen and write at the same time. I'm not saying that the notetaker is hearing what is said but that he is listening as well.

What is the difference between hearing and listening?

Hearing is one directional. You simply hear what is said, allowing some of it to stick, but most of it will be lost within ten to fifteen minutes.

Listening is multidimensional. You are not only hearing but also actually processing the information as you receive it at a much higher level, allowing you to recall it at a later time. Listening requires focus without distraction. You can't listen while you are chatting, playing music in the background, texting, or daydreaming.

Great listeners actually practice three phases: they intently hear what is said, process the information, and prepare a response. This will take practice—even I'm still struggling with being a great listener at all times.

Back to note-taking: I have never been a notetaker, so I don't see any personal value in generating lots of written words that are difficult to interpret after the fact, unless you are exceptional. And there's always one person in the class who can hear, listen, and take notes at the same time. (I suspect that she works twice as hard as the rest of you and is committed to translating her notes after she gets home.)

Taking notes is distracting since we can't write as fast as we speak; therefore, you will always be slightly behind. You also run the risk that you'll misinterpret or write down inaccurate information.

What I would suggest is that you write down "key words" that will serve as memory anchors and reference points for further exploration when preparing for an exam.

Key words (like those used in Bill O'Reilly's "Talking Points Memos") provide a highly reliable way to study and prepare for a lecture or an exam. Your brain is exceptional at recalling information based on key images, numbers, or words. If you don't believe me, watch a few episodes of Discovery Channel's *Brain Games* to glean a better understanding of how your brain operates.

Note-taking is extremely subjective by nature, and you will need to discover for yourself what works best. If all else fails, make friends with the best notetaker in class and ask for a copy just in case.

Stress Management

Let me start by giving you the numero uno advice for every paramedic: only see what you **need** to see.

Your brain is like a thumb drive with finite space limitations before it goes haywire. Every scene, every incident, and every injury and emotion are registered in your brain. If you are not careful with this limited space, your drive will become full, causing you distress and anguish and, in some cases, even posttraumatic stress disorder (PTSD).

Take this advice to heart. I know what you are thinking right now because I thought the same way when I started as a paramedic until someone gave me this same advice.

If you need further proof, speak to some burned-out medics or those who experienced a system overload during the 911 response to the World Trade Center disaster.

Let me take a step back. Stress is not just caused by events at work, whether small or large. Everything and anything can be a cause of stress, especially if you are not in good condition mentally or physically.

In order to manage stress, your relationships, your physical well-being, and your mental health need to be in a positive balance. This requires great self-awareness and a willingness to work on each facet of life. This is truly a life journey as stressors change with age and in different environments.

Since we are all a bit different from one another, no single approach will work for everyone. You will need to discover what works best for you, whether it's religion, meditation, mentorship, counseling, or a distracting hobby. It simply should not be an option for you to neglect finding stress relief and debriefing.

As paramedics, we are a unique bunch of people by nature. We tend to be highly independent, love adrenaline rushes, and work best in short spurts. We don't necessarily like to know more about our patients than the presenting signs and symptoms along with a supporting history to put it all into perspective. This phenomenon is actually a coping mechanism—getting emotionally attached to our patients or families could be stress inducing. Just ask any nurse who works in the critical-care unit. They can handle the patient's care; however, the families' pain and worry and the frequent deaths cause tremendous stress.

Now that we have some perspective, we should discuss some options of stress reduction, both preventative and postevent.

Here are the top five suggestions for stress reduction; however, find something that works for you.

1. Meditation
2. Playing an instrument
3. Distracting hobby such as flying, fishing, etc.
4. Massage therapy
5. Exercise

Commit to doing something that allows your mind to debrief, relax, and free up "bandwidth." You'll find immediate release from your daily stresses. It's a feel-good moment in time but not a fix that will sustain itself indefinitely.

You need to find a rhythm that works for you. For me, I love to fly small airplanes, a hobby that is a complete distracter from my daily stressful jobs. I have to submerge myself in preplanning several days before I go, and when I'm flying, I have stay focused on the task at hand until I safely land my plane once more. Although I fly only once per month on average, I often read articles and blogs and participate in group discussions about flying. Besides flying, I try to meditate daily for at least ten minutes. It centers me and keeps my energy balanced and my thoughts positive. Whenever I feel myself slide to the negative brain, I stop what I'm doing, close the door, shut off the lights, and kick up my feet to meditate for just a few minutes.

It would not do the subject justice to skip over acute stress syndrome, which is often felt immediately after a traumatic experience. This will be different for everyone as our stress threshold differs from person to person. I don't know when it will be your turn, but I do know that all of us have faced such a moment in time.

When you find yourself stressed after an acute event, don't ignore the symptoms of constant thoughts, a guilt complex, visual recall, and at times heart palpitations and hyperventilation. As a paramedic, you will recognize these symptoms but often will have the tendency to disregard them due to fear of being seen as a failure. Too many paramedics have ended their lives because they failed to sound the alarm bells.

It is your duty to keep a watchful eye on your partners and fellow emergency responders. If you feel stressed and overwhelmed after an event, the others are likely feeling it as well. Start a conversation with your supervisor and suggest that your critical-incident stress-debriefing team be dispatched.

When you find yourself in moments of despair, you need to deal with your stress in a safe environment. Reach out to a friend and just talk. Keep telling the story from your perspective, and insert humor if necessary. We have all been there before to some extent or another. Don't become a statistic because of failure to recognize your symptoms or failure to seek assistance.

Life is worth living—call a friend!

National Suicide Prevention Lifeline

1-800-273-8255

Being a *Great* Paramedic Student

I have interacted with hundreds of students over the years and found most to be well intended but ill prepared as paramedic students.

A student by nature is someone who is in the process of learning and development. To learn, one needs to be teachable. This is where you will find the most variability among students.

Lots of students come with just enough knowledge to be dangerous and therefore are not ready to hear, listen, and learn.

To be a *great* student, you need to show respect, listen intently, absorb what is conveyed, acknowledge the information gleaned, and be teachable at all times. This will take effort on your part; however, I can assure you that when these attributes are practiced with great humility, you will receive more than you would have otherwise.

Great students are prepared for each course, class, and shift. They have reviewed materials ahead of time and have formulated relevant questions.

Being a *great* student sounds kind of boring, and it is somewhat predictable. However, your patients' future care is at stake. Do you want the student who got a 65 percent passing grade or the one who got a 90 percent (or above) to take care of you? I know that some of the most brilliant medics are poor test takers, and I also know that they worked twice as hard in the field to learn about their trade and how to apply what they learned.

Whether or not you will be a *great* student is your choice to make. Being a future *Positude* Paramedic requires you to commit the greatest of your efforts in whatever needs to be done.

Getting the Most Out of Your Rotations

This will be your first interaction with medics, nurses, and doctors not directly compensated by your paramedic program. To them, you might be a burden for the day, while others will see you as someone to use as a gofer.

It's time to make an awesome first impression. It all starts by being prepared and arriving on time and never late.

On time = arriving more than fifteen minutes prior to start of your shift

Late = arriving after your start time

Come dressed appropriately and bring proper identification and instruction for your preceptors containing information on what you can and can't do during your rotation. As time progresses, you will be given greater responsibilities and permission to perform certain skills in the field. Make sure you update your preceptor at the beginning of each shift, including the proper signature sheets from your program director.

Your first impression should include giving a short introduction about yourself and a show of appreciation for them acting as your preceptors and sharing their knowledge with you. Speak with confidence and humility and remain teachable at all times.

When completing a ride-along, don't get too comfortable at the beginning of your shift. Take initiative by checking the equipment without being asked to do so. Ask your preceptors pertinent questions, and also ask them to share their experiences.

After completing all of the regular station duties, it's quite all right to sit back, but don't lie down. Show that you are ready to respond as soon as the bell rings. Know before your first call what is expected of you and how you can conform to their workflow, which will differ between preceptors. It all goes back to our four principles of being a *Positude* Paramedic (or paramedic student):

1. Nonnegotiable mutual respect
2. Common bond
3. Common understanding
4. Teachability

Finally, you receive your first opportunity to go on your first 911 call for the day. Be prompt in your response without being overly hasty. Collect your thoughts and start preparing for the call. When you arrive on scene, offer to carry the bags and be the first person after the primary medic to enter the house. At some point in your rotation, you will become the primary responder, with your preceptor now filling the role of coach, mentor, and emergency medic. Regardless, always be the first in the house whenever possible.

At the end of each call and/or shift, debrief with your preceptor. Listen more than you talk; take in the comments whether they seem right or wrong. There's always some truth in every statement. Never argue with your preceptor unless a dangerous situation arises—and at that time you are obligated to say something.

Leave your shift showing gratitude and appreciation. There's no need or any expectation to buy coffee, lunch, or any snacks in between. Great paramedics love to share their thoughts and experiences with students; however, they don't like to be a dentist. (Don't make them pull the information from you.) If you say nothing or do nothing, don't expect them to do something.

Be the positive driving force behind a great experience.

Final Exam

You have reached the point that you have been working toward for the past twelve to twenty-four months. A little stage fright before the final exam is appropriate as it is the culmination of all your learning being tested in one final sitting.

Some of you will just be fine: you have always been great test takers and don't get caught up in the moment. You can essentially skip this section of the book—congrats on reaching your goals.

If you're the opposite kind of student, don't worry. Over the years, I have given advice to students who had great trepidation about sitting for any exam—forget about their final exam. Somehow, you have made it to the end and need to get ready for your final test, but first you need to get your nerves under control.

Using Ativan, pot, and alcohol—although great solutions for quelling nerves—might not be the best way of making it through your exam. However, meditation and relaxation therapy is appropriate but not for everyone.

Let's explore some middle-of-the-road solutions that might work for you.

- Take lots of practice test questions so you know what to expect.
- Identify your weak areas and put in some extra study time.
- Use flash cards to test yourself.
- Convert theory into practice.
- Take a break away from studying and go for a long walk.
- Consult a sports psychologist.

Any of these techniques should be used throughout your career if test taking causes you great anxiety.

4

Strategy 4: Finding the Right Job

Congrats, you have passed your final exam, and now it's time to find the right job for you. Emergency services, especially EMS, are hierarchical by nature; therefore, it's likely that you will need to start as a transport paramedic. Depending on your determination, you can progress through the systems pretty quickly. If necessary, you might need to move around a little until you get into a position of your liking.

Below, I will outline my personal viewpoint on each of the jobs highlighted. At some point in my career I have been in each of these roles, and with a few I have learned enough to provide you a glimpse of what the jobs are like. My goal is for you to get a sense of the different opportunities you have as a paramedic.

Transport Paramedic

Some might see this as an entry-level position into paramedicine; however, a *Positude* Paramedic will see this as the opportunity of a lifetime. Don't get caught up in the stigma of "only 911 medics are real medics." Nonsense! Every paramedic has an essential role to play in our health-care system and emergency services.

Being a transport paramedic allows you to grow and broaden your experience base in multiple settings. Actually, I can argue that some of the sickest patients in our nursing homes are treated and cared for by transport paramedics. Our oath to do no harm is equal for all patients, regardless of how they activated the system. Each patient deserves only the very best. Therefore, as a transport paramedic, your job is equally important as all the others.

The main difference between a transport and 911 paramedic is the fact that a transport paramedic has scheduled pickups for appointments at doctor's offices, dialysis centers, and many other locations.

This is your opportunity to develop excellent customer service skills and to sharpen your patient assessment skills.

As a transport paramedic, you will frequently be called upon for interfacility transport—transferring patients to a higher level of care. In the next section, I will delve into the job of the critical-care paramedic; however, as a transport paramedic, you are frequently thrust into the same role without the extra training. The key factor to your success as a transport paramedic is to be prepared for the unknown, which is true for every one of these positions. You have to know your equipment and supplies inside and out: its location, function, how to troubleshoot it, and how to apply it to your patients.

Regardless of position, you still have to remain prepared at all times to jump into action on the 911 side of emergency services. Mutual aid for the transport divisions across our country is not an uncommon occurrence, especially where volunteer services remain the primary responder.

On a personal note, some of my sincerest interactions with our elderly population, especially extremely coherent ninety-plus-year-olds, have provided some enlightening moments I would not trade for anything. Our old folks still have lots to offer to us young folks.

Lastly, it is perfectly all right if you choose to be a transport paramedic for the remainder of your working years: the key is "right people, right role," as Jim Collins describes in *Good to Great*.

Critical-Care Paramedic (CCP)

This is a great progressive step for any paramedic to get a better understanding of the technical complexities of interfacility critical-care transport.

Though CCP has not yet become the new standard of care for critical-care transport, it should be in the near future with the availability of certified critical-care courses throughout the country.

A critical-care transport of a patient with complex trauma or medical conditions is not just another transport. Many moons ago, it was not uncommon for a critical-care nurse or respiratory care technician to join you on the transfer, and on rare occasions even a doctor would join you.

Today, a critical-care paramedic is asked to handle such situations on his own or with the assistance from another paramedic or EMT. That is a heavy burden and an awesome responsibility that should not be taken lightly.

I would highly recommend that *all* paramedics become certified critical-care paramedics. Continuing education is a vital part of being a *Positude* Paramedic; you should never stop learning and exploring.

There are few things more exciting than transporting a patient to a higher level of care while managing the ventilator, five to six drips, the cardiac monitor, and a chest tube or two. This will have you sitting on the edge of your seat and will give you a great sense of accomplishment after you've transferred care to a team of doctors and nurses at the receiving facility.

911 Paramedic

Under most circumstances, as a 911 paramedic you are dedicated to the 911 system, which means that responses are generated from emergency requests. Most often, you are dispatched by a central command or municipality dispatch center or police department.

911 paramedics travel in a variety of vehicles, including fly-cars, ambulances, motorcycles, bicycles, or on foot. Your primary function is to provide emergency care ranging from a small scrape to penetrating trauma, abdominal pain to a cardiac arrest.

911 paramedics need to have a great sense of community, partnership, relationship building, and situational awareness. You truly never know what you are going to run into next.

In our larger population centers, 911 medics respond in a multitiered system whereby either police or fire services, or both, also respond to assist in rendering care and transferring the patients to an awaiting ambulance.

We can't underestimate the hazardous situations 911 medics need to operate in. Don't ever take for granted your personal security and safety. Police officers' responsibilities at medical/traumatic emergencies are to ensure that the scene is safe and to provide emergency care until the 911 medic arrives. Factually speaking, most of our 911 medics are only backed up by police officers if the situation warrants requiring a whole other level of situational awareness.

As a 911 medic, you need to be prepared for the unknown, work closely with your partners in care, and have the ability to prioritize emergency care. You will often find yourself in the back of the ambulance with total strangers who might or might not wear a patch identifying their level of training. Don't be shocked if they tell you that they have been an EMT for only a month or only ride a few hours per month. This will take special patience on your part. It's time to be a lifesaver, coach, mentor, teacher, and emotional supporter all at the same time. It's actually an interesting part of our job.

For you who are interested in working in large metropolitan areas where 911 medics work for the city, you will have to be less concerned about the volunteers and more heavily focused on the physical condition and the often less-than-pleasant environments you will have to work in. You will most likely have graduated from the agency's paramedic program, which should have prepared you for what is coming your way. My message to you is to be vigilant with managing your stress and identifying signs or symptoms of burnout syndrome. You will be very busy day or night with few support systems, subsisting on a diet that is not even suitable for a hyena, and lacking proper rest—these conditions will push the best of us over the edge if we are not preemptive in managing our physical and mental health needs.

Being a 911 medic can also be lots of fun and exciting, especially when you take specialty assignments such as concerts, street fairs, beach patrols, special operations, or movie sets. Each will allow you to see emergency services through a different prism, and I highly recommend that you sign up for some of these events as a stress reducer and break from your everyday assignment.

Being a 911 medic is truly a privilege. The public puts a tremendous amount of trust in your ability to serve them with the highest standard of care. Live up to these standards at all times. As 911 medics are the most visible of all paramedics, it is your duty to carry forward with great professionalism and a positive attitude or *positude*.

Flight Paramedic

This is literally a three-dimensional job. It's considered the most advanced position a paramedic can function in today. If you can overcome the fear of flying in a fixed-wing or rotor-wing plane, this position is a great goal to set for yourself. It's an awesome opportunity to work at the top of your license and learn more about neonatal, pediatric, medical, and trauma care than you have up to this point in time.

Besides the clinical care, there are two other people you will need to learn to partner with and work with in great unison. Your pilot literally has your life in his hands each time you fly. It's paramount that you spend time studying aviation and truly become a partner in flight, not just to provide clinical care but to assist your pilot in the flight itself. You will be an extra set of eyes in the skies looking for obstacles or other flying objects. You will learn to operate the radios, GPS, and emergency procedures just in case an engine fails. You can't just pull off to the side of the road to check for a flat tire. It's a tremendous responsibility—take this into consideration if you want to make being a flight medic one of your professional goals.

In contrast with being a 911 medic, where your partner is another EMT or paramedic, as a flight medic your second partner will most likely be a nurse. Although he or she has received training in EMS, the nurse's core strength is taking care of critically ill patients who need transport from one hospital intensive care unit (ICU) to another ICU that has a higher level of care. I will say that competition for flight nurse positions is so fearsome that most applicants are paramedics who went back to school to become registered nurses. Regardless of their background, you will need to learn to partner with someone in a very different environment from being on the street. You will learn so much from each other, and if you get the balance right, you will work off each other's strengths and weaknesses.

On a personal note, I had the honor to be a flight medic from 2003 to 2008 with *STAT* Flight out of Westchester Medical Center, New York. I've included some of my personal experiences of being a flight medic in the one hundred experience stories later in the book. Although I love being a 911 medic after twenty-four years, I still think that being a flight medic was the epitome of my paramedic career. As a private pilot myself, it brought together the sciences I care for most: medicine, aviation, navigation, stress management, critical care, and nursing.

If you have the opportunity and drive to spend many hours studying and completing rotations in neonatal intensive care units (NICU), pediatric intensive care units (PICU), trauma intensive care units (TICU), and ICUs, I encourage you to make this your ten-year goal. You won't be paid much, but it is an experience of a lifetime.

I have nothing but fond memories of every flight except two where I was so nauseated that all I wanted to do was land safely and never fly again (until my next shift, of course).

Special acknowledgments to those I served with as a flight medic from day one: Chrissie, Rich, and TJ, you will always be part of my greatest memories. Bill Palmer, who was my favorite crankiest pilot: I miss you every day. Bill Pope, my low-flying pilot with fantastic perspective. David Lichtbach, the forever bachelor until you found Miss Right and all the fantastic flying stories. Jenna, Dave, Maura, Elena, Ken, Sam, and many more great flight nurses—I learned so much from you.

Fire Medic

This is one area I know the least about. I will provide some basic information for you to explore, but I encourage you to do some additional research if this is one of your primary goals (and is available in your geographic area).

As a paramedic student at Hudson Valley Community College in 1993, I completed my ride-alongs with Troy Fire Department Medic 3, stationed out of the central office in downtown Troy, New York.

I don't recall their names, but I remember them well—rough, strong-looking guys, the quintessential firefighters. They were the nicest guys you could ever meet and were very supportive in furthering my learning as a paramedic student.

Although they saw themselves primarily as firefighters, they were cross-trained to become paramedics to provide primary first response in the city of Troy, which had contracted Mohawk Ambulance to transport patients to the hospital. I believe that this arrangement came about due to pure economics. As fire safety improved, call volume dwindled. Adding the responsibility of EMS to the duties of firefighters increased their volume substantially since it justified maintaining the size of the department.

On rare occasions, you may see a similar model in a local police department. I find this a bit of an odd relationship in being a medic and a cop at the same time; however, I'm a big proponent of police officers learning to provide emergency care, including administering Narcan, EpiPens, and CPAP, especially in areas where it could take ten or more minutes for a paramedic response.

You can see the similarities between the two professions and the reasoning for why they have been mixed into one. As someone considering entering emergency services, you should investigate all options available, including not only hourly pay but also the benefit packages offered by each.

Most often, fire service is a third service that is offered by the local municipalities as required by law. Although it's likely to be a civil service, the pay and fringe benefits (including a twenty- to twenty-five-year retirement package) are much better than those offered by services other than the fire or police services.

If you happen to live in parts of the country where this setup is the norm, make a phone call to the local rescue station and request to meet the chief. He or she will gladly tell you all about the services the station provides and the benefits of joining a service where fire medics are standard.

Community Paramedic

This is truly a pioneering area for paramedicine. It's our greatest opportunity to expand the role of paramedicine in our communities and to provide an alternative for those who can no longer work as transport or 911 medics due to injuries, fatigue, or age but who are not ready to hang up their stethoscopes.

Since there's no standard curriculum in place for this type of program (besides some large-scale pilot programs mostly in the more rural areas of the country), I will take the liberty to describe the future of community paramedicine from my perspective.

Growing up in Holland, we had a community nurse who assisted the elderly with wound care, basic physical therapy, bathing, blood-pressure checks, blood sugar checks, and blood tests to regulate index medications. This model still exists today in some parts of Holland and is actually making a strong comeback. In the United States, we deploy home-care nurses such as visiting nurse services (VNS) to provide these types of services, but only for patients who qualify for this level of care, most often after a hospital discharge. Although this service is available through private nursing agencies as well, it comes at a considerable cost to the patient.

Speaking from experience, community paramedics should not compete with nurses over the same patients to prevent extended litigation between nursing unions that may oppose the role of the community paramedics.

Community paramedics need to position themselves as "physician extenders," similar to what their role is in emergency services, but instead of reporting to the emergency-room directors, they report to a primary-care provider. Prehospital visits are a vital component of population health management, whereby a community paramedic is charged with frequent short visits to patients' homes to take blood pressure, do blood work, and to assess the home for obvious safety hazards. If necessary, these visits can be followed up with a more complex assessment by VNS.

Beyond regularly scheduled short appointments (fewer than twenty minutes per patient), patients can call community paramedics for minor emergencies instead of going to a high-cost urgent-care facility or emergency department for care. Community paramedics can be taught to do minor stitching, wound care, and assessment for flu/colds/fevers, and can consult the primary-care physician via telemedicine if necessary.

I believe that community paramedicine would be an exciting opportunity for paramedics to transition into, and collectively we can bring down the cost of health care significantly if this was deployed nationwide.

Long-Term Goals Postparamedicine

Most of you, but not all of you, will pursue additional education past your paramedic degree. It is our hope that someday paramedicine will become a true career choice that allows each of you to provide a decent living for your families without the need to work eighty hours per week, like most of you do.

In actuality, paramedicine has gone from a certificate to an associate's degree program in most states. Our goal should be to set the standards higher—to the level of a bachelor's degree at minimum—with opportunities to advance.

Today, that is still just a dream. However, there are some bright folks around the country working on advancing our profession to the next level. Even better days are still ahead of us.

In this section, we are going to assume that you are a paramedic or soon will be a paramedic; however, you will only use this as a transition to a career.

Although I still work full-time nights as a paramedic, I too felt the need to go back to school to get my BS in economics and MBA in executive management and have since become a board-certified Fellow of the American College of Healthcare Executives (ACHE).

Many of my friends have done the same—very successfully, I might say. Some are now nurses, physician assistants, emergency-room doctors and directors, health-care administrators, and successful entrepreneurs. I'm also pretty sure that most will tell you that being a paramedic was pretty awesome, and most of them continue to work as medics at special events or per diem.

Let this be a guiding light for you. Being a paramedic is pretty awesome and a truly fulfilling profession where you can be the difference between life and death.

Here are a handful of career opportunities where your paramedic experience will come in very handy:

- Registered nurse (RN)
- Physician assistant (PA) or doctor
- Emergency services (fire/police/EMS)
- Emergency management (federal/state/local)
- Health-care administration
- Education

You will have a leg up on the other students in your class if you are a paramedic, especially if you have a couple years of experience under your belt.

Most of these career choices above have limited space in their programs, so having your paramedic certificate might be the edge you need to be selected.

Being a paramedic will significantly improve your critical thinking skills; your ability to assess patients in their home setting; and most importantly, your interviewing skills, which are a vital part of your future career as a medic, RN, PA, or doctor.

If for nothing else, you have the ability to earn a few extra dollars while finishing your degrees by working as a paramedic on the side.

I'm a true believer that all paramedics should continue to learn and explore opportunities as they relate to the field of medicine. Your patients will be the beneficiaries of your learning.

Part II:

Five Skills

5

Skill 1: Partnerships

Communication Skills

You know what the top three reasons are for why failures occur? Lack of effective communication, communication, and communication. We cannot overemphasize the importance of good communication in patient safety and teamwork.

We discussed the difference between listening and hearing in chapter 3. Kindly refer back to it one more time before you proceed.

Communication skills include both verbal and nonverbal communication. Often, we say things but our words are not clearly understood. If you proceed without clarification, it increases the likelihood of a poor outcome or decrease in efficiency.

Other times, we give a look or posture that sends a message without us saying a word. This too can lead to misinterpretation and failures.

As a paramedic, the majority of your career will be spent with a partner who is either an EMT or another paramedic. You will need to become a highly effective communicator, especially as it relates to patient care and maintaining situational awareness.

Over time, if you make a real effort, you will learn to communicate without ever saying a word to each other. You can anticipate each other's next action, question, or need. This will take time to develop, and much of this is done through trial and error.

Since communication skills are so vital to quality care, supervisors need to be sensitive when scheduling shifts. Whenever possible, partners should be kept together unless there's a true lack of chemistry between them.

Great paramedics learn to listen mindfully while playing the support role in a particular scenario. They will be able to anticipate their partner's next move and need.

In time, you will be able to finish each other's sentences. If you have any doubt about this phenomenon, just ask some old-timers. They will likely tell you that they don't need to say much when working in true partnership, especially during critical calls.

I won't leave you hanging by not giving you something to think about. There are two key factors to great communication:

1. You need to develop a strong common bond and common understanding when working with a partner: for example, you need to decide who will take the lead on the first job, who will go to the hospital with the patient, who will drive, whose turn is it to intubate the patient, and so on. Each of these actions will require a slightly different setup as you leave your station to respond.

2. You need to remain teachable at all times, especially if you work with different partners. Each person brings a unique perspective to managing emergencies; therefore, you will need to adjust your style from time to time. More importantly,

being adaptable or nimble allows you to learn what skills over time will make you a better paramedic.

Building Vital Partnerships

As mentioned before, you will be spending significant time with a partner over the span of your career.

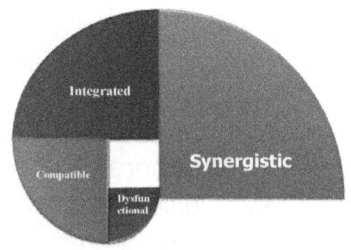

It will take real work on your part to make sure that your relationships are not just functional but rather fully synergistic. There are two fundamental areas that will allow you to break down barriers and bring your partnership to the next level of performance. This works much better, of course, if you get to work with the same partners often. However, these principles hold true for any relationship or partnership as well.

Getting to Know Them

Make time to get to know your partners a bit better by showing interest in their personal lives, families, children, and hobbies. This will establish a bond of care and an emotional commitment between you. It will also improve your ability to communicate more effectively.

Understanding Them

Your goal is to become truly synergistic with your partner, which will require you to not only know them but to understand them.

This is equally important whether you work with the same partner each shift or with someone different each day.

Many of your partners will have alpha personalities, which will require some adjustments to prevent conflict between you.

Great medics know when to lead and when to be led. You will learn about this the hard way, most likely.

As you make a real effort to get to know your partners, allow them to lead on the first few calls and you will have time to adjust.

Furthermore, use the exercise below to develop a strong synergistic relationship with your partner. You are looking to strengthen each other's weaknesses and produce the best outcomes. This will take time and work on your part.

Tool Kit #3

Expanded Exercises

Step 1	Step 2		Step 3	Step 4	
Name	Determine the Level of Partnership		Status Build, Maintain, Repair, Distance	Next Steps	
	Current	Desired		Plan	Completion Date

Critical Feedback

I frequently use an equation to explain the magic of performance if both technical skill and behavioral capacity are maximized.

Performance = (Technical Skills × Behavioral Capacity)

After years of training and developing your skills, you will be able to perform skills in your sleep. This is an unlikely failure point unless you become complacent. Complacency is a behavior or lack of awareness; it doesn't mean you don't know how to perform the technical skill.

Lack of behavioral capacity or being not optimized is a personal choice. However, you need to be aware of your attitude and emotions before you can start optimizing your actual behavior.

Since most of us neither are too critical of ourselves nor are likely to address negative performance with our peers, you will need to learn to both receive and provide critical feedback.

Feedback is your greatest ally in becoming a great paramedic. You need to hear from your partners, supervisors, volunteers, and even your patients.

To make it truly meaningful, you need to make time and put real effort into this exercise.

Stress Debriefing

I'm going to address stress debriefing in multiple sections of this book because I want to drive home the importance of both stress management (prevention) and stress debriefing (postincident).

In a strong partnership, it is your responsibility to keep an eye on your partner's mental well-being both before and after an incident. Don't take this responsibility for granted or think that you know your partners well enough to not pay extra attention.

I have experienced some losses of very close friends and coworkers over the years and felt a level of guilt postevent where I questioned myself—had I done enough?

I'm not sure who came up with this, but it's something that each of us should employ. Reach Out Wednesday is a set time to make a caring call to your current or past partners. See how they are doing, ask them if they want to talk about something, or just simply tell them that you care.

I practice this each and every shift, and it certainly goes both ways. Some of my partners might say that I need to debrief more often than the other way around. Briefing or debriefing is just like how teaching is learning. You get to know each other a bit more and de-stress at the same time.

Next time you work, ask your partner how he or she is doing. Next time you finish a hot job, slow down for a minute or two to talk about it together. Make a phone call the next morning to see how he or she is doing after a good night's sleep (or not).

Make sure you don't forget about yourself—there's nothing more important than your mental health. If you ignore it, you will get burned out at some point in time. It will lead to poor quality of care and ultimately safety lapses that could actually hurt someone.

Don't be too proud to ask for assistance.

6

Skill 2: Situational Awareness

Safety First

What are the three most likely failure points that result in poor clinical outcomes?

1. Failure to communicate
2. Failure to communicate
3. Failure to communicate

What are the three most likely failure points that result in injuries on the job?

1. Safety violations
2. Safety violations
3. Safety violations

As a paramedic or health-care provider, you have to make personal safety of paramount importance, the cornerstone of your professional career. You should never compromise your safety to provide for others unless risk exposures are calculated and mitigated to the greatest possible extent.

You will find yourself in highly emotionally driven situations, and you will be tempted to act on instinct rather than rational thought. This could potentially lead to injury to yourself or others.

We have all been there. I remember one day on the thruway jumping into a burning car to pull the driver to safety. It was a risky, purely adrenaline-driven action that I took without due regard for my own safety. It was heroic and stupid at the same time.

I'm admonishing you to raise awareness in difficult situations and, whenever possible, to assess your personal safety before acting.

Being Aware of Your Surroundings

Did you know that adrenaline actually causes tunnel vision?

Your heart starts racing, your mind starts going, and you act on instinct and feel hyperfocused on the task at hand.

It also causes you to miss the little things in your peripheral vision that could be the difference between life and death.

Tunnel vision can also be the cause of complacency or lack of caring—a "been there, done that" kind of an attitude.

Even the most prepared and mindful paramedics can tell you their stories where they failed to look at the bigger picture, situations that could potentially have had a negative impact.

I distinctively remember a scenario when I was responding to another hypoglycemic call in a quiet upstate community. Although I knew that these types of patients are a bit unpredictable and had prepared for that, I was not prepared to find a .44 Magnum under her pillow while patient was waking up (after we had administered D50 to her). Luckily, all went well; however, this could have ended up as a tragedy of unknown proportions if the confused hypoglycemic patient had thought that we were intruders.

Always be aware and mindful of your surroundings, and don't assume that the very old or the very young can't cause havoc.

Think of the unthinkable without being paranoid. Keep your eyes wide open, and in large scenes ask or assign someone the role of keeping an eye on the larger picture.

Your sole objective is to provide excellence in care and go home to your family at night.

Emergency Response

We are all little kids inside, still running toward the sirens or at least wondering what is going on.

Did you know that the most dangerous portion of responding to an emergency is when you're driving Code 3? It is often an adrenaline-filled event that requires a hyperawareness of surroundings and anticipating the moves of all drivers on the road.

For years, especially early on in my career, I truly believed that the faster I drove, the better the clinical outcomes. I really got lucky on many occasions by not crashing and hurting myself or others on the road.

Studies have shown that a Code 3 response is merely a few minutes faster at best and poses a potential significant cost. Is it really worth life or limb to drive like a bat out of hell?

An emergency response needs to be carefully measured against your capabilities, the time of the day, the road conditions, the seriousness of the call, and many other factors.

When you buy a new or used car, you go for a test ride to see how well it accelerates, brakes, or if it has certain tendencies when rounding corners. Make sure you do the same when you start driving an emergency vehicle. Be warned that ambulances are top heavy and rather unstable at higher speeds, leaving them vulnerable in high winds and going around tight corners.

Every emergency response should be measured and executed with safety in mind. If you can't get there in one piece, you won't do any good for your patients.

Incident Command

When does an event become an incident? It all depends on the resources required to mitigate the situation. In some communities, this might be an accident involving a few cars, while in a larger community an "incident" might have to involve multiple departments responding.

Regardless of the situation, only one person should be in charge, or you chance failure. Let's be a little less dramatic in terms of failure; however, efficiency is lost if too many people are in charge and potentially the timeliness of treatment and transport can be reduced as well.

As a *Positude* Paramedic, you will need to learn the structure of command and control. It comes directly from our military partners, and this is the only case when I'm highly supportive of directive leadership.

In planning, mitigation, and preparedness, incident commanders need to be inclusive and collaborative, and all participants need to be creative and engaged. At the time of a response, it is paramount that you as a responding paramedic respect the command structure and follow orders to the greatest extent possible without compromising personal, team, or patient safety.

If you are ever selected, assigned, or volunteered to be the incident commander, practice communicating with great clarity and strive for common understanding and common purpose among all responders. To be successful, surround yourself with the right people and put them in the right positions.

This will require additional study beyond what you have or will receive in your paramedic education.

Emergency Management

Although I separated the discussion about incident command from emergency management, they are synonymous. You really can't have one without the other.

As an aspiring *Positude* Paramedic, you will be playing an important element in any emergency you respond to, especially when you are the first responder.

Although I'm not going to explain in great detail what the incident command system (ICS) is or does, I'm going to provide a glimpse of its role and impact in the overall management of an incident. I strongly encourage you to seek further information and, whenever possible, to participate as a responder in local drills. If you really want a unique perspective, play a mock patient in the next drill. It will give you a renewed respect for both the provider and the patient.

The ICS system was developed many moons ago by the fire service after a large-scale wildfire in California. Multiple services' responders pushed the fire around without coordinating between the services, causing many acres to be scorched. It was not until after the fact when all the responding agencies came together that they realized that they could have done better—actually much better.

After much discussion, they all agreed on creating a single command structure. This command would provide instruction to the front lines, and front-line officers would provide feedback to the incident commander so he or she could make decisions.

After years of learning and refining this system at real-life events, the ICS system was created and has now become a widely accepted response method for managing a large-scale event.

7

Skill 3: Patient Assessment

Introduction

I wish I was wrong, but I'm afraid I am not. Without painting all the paramedic programs with a broad stroke, 80 percent of our recent graduates are not prepared to perform a solid and comprehensive patient assessment.

Patient assessment starts from the second you receive the request for response. Generally, a *Positude* Paramedic will gather intelligence through each phase of response, treatment, transport, and transfer of care in the receiving hospital.

Over the next few pages as I discuss Skill Three: Patient Assessment, I encourage you to reassess the way you deliver care today and challenge yourself to adapt and adjust continuously. Only practice makes (near) perfect.

You are never too old to learn new behaviors or unlearn bad ones that could potentially prevent you from being a *Positude* Paramedic. I'm not telling what to do or even telling you what is best; I'm asking you to assess and reassess your current behaviors and to make adjustments as necessary.

Relate; don't compare.

Creating a Safe Environment

Part of the reason I chose to be a paramedic is the fact that you never know what you are going to see or do or where you're going to go next. It's an exciting opportunity to see patients in their natural environments. Maybe that makes it sound like the patients are animals in their "natural habitat." However, there's real value to seeing patients in their home and to have the ability to look in their refrigerator and cabinets and to see the way they dress, sleep, and relax.

It is equally important to inspect the interior of an upside-down car or a crunched-up bike or motorcycle.

Your intuition and experiences will allow you to draw conclusions or develop working diagnoses that can lead to better decision-making processes, care, and clinical outcomes.

Having said this, none of this can or should be done unless you are working in a safe environment. This is not an assessment to make postevent or after an injury has occurred.

Make it your absolute priority to always think and consider safety before proceeding or rushing forward. As a paramedic, make it your responsibility to raise your situational awareness, slow down, and proceed when it is safe to do so.

Don't give in to peer pressure to proceed when your intuition tells you to slow down. It is your responsibility to provide care to your patients in a safe environment and not create additional injuries by taking undue risk.

Asking the Right Questions

Over my many years of working as a paramedic, flight medic, and health-care administrator who frequently makes rounds at the patient's bedside, I truly believe that the "patient interview" is a lost art.

How do you know when to ask what, how to ask, what not to say or ask, what to tell or not to tell? How do you verify and confirm? There are lots of great questions and, in my opinion, too few answers.

I'm going to attempt to outline a skill that most paramedics, including myself, need to strengthen.

As a senior medic, it is my responsibility to ensure that these skills are passed on to the next generation, especially now that our EMTs walk onto the scene with a touchpad computer to electronically document demographics. It drives me completely bananas.

I accept the future and the use of electronics, but nothing is more important than making contact with your patients in an empathic manner and not hiding behind a computer, tablet, or PDA.

Now that I'm done pontificating, let's transition to what a great interview with your patients could look like.

It all starts at the time someone calls 911 or places a request for emergency transport, triggering a paramedic response.

Listen carefully to the dispatch information to get a sense of the urgency, a description of the illness or injury, use of technical jargon versus plain-spoken words, and any updates along the way. The dispatch is your first paragraph of your patient interview, requiring you to remain open minded and teachable at the same time.

It's a difficult subject but the one we need to review for a few minutes: your personal hygiene. Your patient will open up to you if you are approachable, look professional, and don't look or smell offensive.

I'm not going to judge you on your personal habits. Instead, I'm going to deplore you to be sensitive to your partners and especially your patients. There is no place for bad body odor from smoking or not applying deodorant—you have full control over this and should make a real effort to prevent such a scenario.

Looking and acting like a *Positude* Paramedic is your responsibility so that you will carry our profession to the next level of performance and recognition. Make this a priority for yourself.

Finally, when you arrive on the scene, if you are going to run this call, you should be the first to arrive at your patient's side. As you enter, make an announcement and introduce yourself by clearly stating your name and asking the patient how he or she would like to be addressed. You have established your first contact and, more importantly, your first impression.

Right at that moment, your patient has formed an opinion of you, and this will determine how the rest of the conversation will go.

What you do next greatly varies between individuals, and it really depends on how tall/big you are and the location of the patient. As a six-foot-five medic, I have to be conscious of my tallness and how overpowering that can feel to a patient who is lying down, sitting, or at times even standing.

When possible, bring yourself to your patient's eye level before you start your interview, preserving your and the patient's personal space. Always ask yourself, "How would I feel in this scenario as a patient?" It is a great barometer to use to gauge your approach.

As you start the patient interview portion of your assessment, transition to being a great listener. Pick up on every symptom that is described that represents a small piece of the puzzle. Some puzzles are easy to solve, while others are more complex or simply perplexing.

Let the patient tell the story without too many interruptions but ask for clarification as necessary. Be mindful and maintain an index of suspicion, especially whenever a present family member is overbearing or telling you a story that doesn't fit the physical presentation of the patient.

As you collect evidence, don't get ahead of yourself or inadvertently create tunnel vision by prematurely making up your mind about a diagnosis. Collect *all* information and verify with your patient that you have understood correctly.

Even the very best interviewers will from time to time learn something new upon arrival at the hospital when the receiving medical staff starts asking questions. Don't feel bad—it happens to all of us.

When we see our patients, the situation is often mayhem and thus nerve-racking for them, which makes it difficult for our patients to remember less relevant details. Because of this phenomenon, it is even more important for you to ask the right questions to get accurate responses.

Practice makes perfect, or at least it improves the likelihood that you'll get enough answers to develop a working diagnosis and from there start a treatment plan.

Head-to-Toe Exam

I sometimes wonder if millennials are really less connected emotionally or physically due to oversaturation and exposure to electronics and social media, which prevents them from connecting with their patients.

It might just be that I have gotten older and have forgotten about my own skills when I first became a paramedic.

Regardless of the truth in the matter, we need to do a better job in educating and teaching all medics the benefits of a great head-to-toe exam.

I strongly encourage all of you to go back to basics and learn to perform a thorough head-to-toe exam, starting by observing your patient in the environment in which she was found. Use all of your senses, even if it's less than pleasant.

Your nose is a powerful tool in your investigatory process since it can pick up odors that are linked to infections, alcohol, or blood. Your eyes can observe the organization of personal belongings and the general environment. Your ears can pick up sounds that your patient is making, and your fingertips can pick up temperature, textures, and moisture levels that will tell you more than you will ever see.

It's all about the *skin*! It's not only your largest organ but also is affected by most illnesses, whether it's a fever, sepsis, shock, dysrhythmias, or fainting spells. Learn and study the power of the skin—you will be a much better *Positude* Paramedic because of it.

Another lost art is percussion and auscultation of the lungs, heart, liver, and abdominal cavity. So much can be learned by listening first and percussing before palpating all quadrants. Seek out a professional or even take a course to learn about these vital skills.

Last but not least are your extremities. What can we possibly learn from touching, feeling, palpating, observing, and moving your patient's extremities? One thing is for sure: you can check for motor, neuro, and sensory functions—although it is difficult to assess these against a baseline if this is your first interaction with this particular patient.

Hold your patient's hand and feel her grip, sense a tremor, and look at her dorsal hand veins when level with the heart or above her head.

All these little nuances found during a completed head-to-toe examination will assist you in making a better working diagnosis and treatment plan.

Nonverbal Communication

Now that we are done with interviewing your patient and have inspected every square inch of her body, what else could possibly be left for us to do?

Did you ever study "body language" in high school, college, or in your paramedic course? If not, you should. The power of observation is truly amazing in learning more about your patient's condition.

Watch how she breathes; observe how she walks, talks, drinks, or eats; and also, notice what she drinks or eats. Is she making eye contact or avoiding your gaze? Is she fiddling around or quietly staring out of the window? Are her arms closed, hugging her chest tightly, or is her posture open, shoulders back, with an easy smile on her faces?

Nonverbal communication is as powerful, if not more so, than verbal communication in many scenarios. Be mindful of your mindfulness, and take time to observe the entire body throughout the emergency—it will allow you to see things that otherwise would go unnoticed.

Each Assessment Tells a Story

Utilizing the best of your skills, you will quickly see that both your observations/findings during the interview and the patient's physical presentation are making sense together, allowing you to see a diagnosis with clarity and optimizing the patient's care. This will lead to better clinical outcomes.

It truly is a game of connecting the dots. You have to determine whether it's:

- Chest pain: muscular versus cardiac
- Kidney stones versus gallbladder attack
- Cerebrovascular accident (CVA) versus transient ischemic attack (TIA)
- Compensation shock versus decompensated shock
- Bacterial versus viral infections
- Placenta abruptio versus placenta previa
- Grand mal seizure versus petit mal seizure
- Asthma versus congestive heart failure

I could name many more scenarios to make my point. If you have command over your situational awareness and your interviewing and physical assessment skills, you will likely be able to develop a differential diagnosis by connecting the dots. It will take practice and a deep knowledge of systems to hone your skills, but failure to learn and develop these skills could potentially lead to making bad decisions and poor clinical outcomes.

A *Positude* Paramedic will be on a lifetime journey of learning and developing, and you owe it to your patients to put in the work.

8

Skill 4: Patient Care

With Skills 1–3 firmly in your grip, I'm going to transition to discuss some very specific tools, strategies, and technical skills that will assist you both in making differential diagnoses as well as in treatments. I have highlighted just a vital few that are most important on critical-care calls.

There are two distinctive categories of response, each of which requires a different mind-set—although your personal safety should be assessed in both scenarios.

Let's discuss medical emergencies first since they will make up 80 percent or more of your call volume. In reality, only about 2 percent of all your responses require your critical-care skills such as intubation, CPEP, cardiac resuscitation, or medication management.

Over time and with experience, you will see from the moment you make contact which patients are going to fit into this category. However, your ability to take care of your patients doesn't only depend on your skills at their bedside; it all depends on your level of preparation and familiarity with your equipment and technology, which will assist you in making the right decisions and providing the right therapies.

Below I have listed the top five skills you need to master as soon as possible. Knowing and understanding each of these tools is going to be the difference between life and death at some point in time.

Did you know that most people who use technology like smartphones only know about and use 10 percent of its capabilities? It's not much different in regard to the use of ventilators, IV pumps, 12-lead EKGs, or End-Tidal CO_2 monitors.

As a *Positude* Paramedic, you should be able to fully operate or apply each piece of equipment in pitch-black darkness without having to search for adjuncts or roaming through menu screens, trying to find the right mode. Make it your business to know your stuff inside and out.

Learn about the relationship between room air SaO_2 and O_2 administration or the significance of wave forms during assisted ventilations. Learn the range of End-Tidal CO_2 during an intubation attempt; know when to stop to ventilate before it is too late. I can go on and on, but this handbook is not meant to be a teaching tool for medical management of a patient but rather to reinforce how urgent it is for you to study and never stop learning about disease management or the capabilities of your tools.

Medical Emergencies
- Pulse oximetry
- Airway management
- End-Tidal CO_2
- Blood pressure
- 12-Lead EKGs

Although some medical emergencies such as abdominal aortic aneurism (AAA) or GI bleeds feel more like a trauma call, most traumatic emergencies will have a distinctive feel to them. It's likely to be outside—in a workplace, roadway, or anywhere in between. It will likely involve distracting injuries such as fractures, abrasions, and lacerations.

Each trauma call will require your very best focus in communication, situational awareness, connecting the dots, and providing expedient care in a safe setting.

It's also more likely to affect your judgment due to the sudden adrenaline rush from going to a hot job. Some paramedics are affected by this more than others.

As you will learn in Advanced Trauma Life Support (ATLS), time is of the essence. The golden hour remains the target: to get a patient from the scene into an operating room theater within sixty minutes of the incident. Therefore, as a paramedic, you need to be hyperaware of the ticking clock and continuously reestablish the sense of urgency. Time is tissue!

Over the past twenty years, only two treatment protocols have changed drastically. We used to backboard everybody and administer lots of fluids en route to the hospital. Today, only some patients should be boarded or given significant amounts of fluids. Know and understand the difference: your patients' comfort and survivability will depend on it.

Lastly and maybe most importantly, know when to apply a tourniquet and when to decompress a chest. Each can be done safely if the injury doesn't require you to do so; however, the opposite can't be said. Failure to recognize a pneumothorax or tension pneumothorax or arterial bleeding from an extremity will lead to devastating outcomes. You will rarely use these skills, if ever, but when you need them, it will be the difference between life and death. Stay on top of your game by frequently simulating these kinds of emergencies. Your patients depend on your skills.

9

Skill 5: Medication Management

The vast majority of your responses will not require you to administer medication, but when you do have to intervene, you need to be very comfortable with knowing what to do, when to do it, and how it is going to affect the patient.

You will spend lots of time in class studying pharmacology and will use your short-term memory to get passing grades. However, postgraduation, you will spend very little time reviewing, discussing, or even using the medications you are authorized to carry.

Besides the medications in your first-response equipment, you will need to have working knowledge of common vitamins, herbal medications, and prescriptions. It sounds overwhelming, and it is.

It is impossible for you to know them all; therefore, it is even more important for you to learn about the dozens of resources that are available to assist you in managing medications.

I'm going to delve into three topics that you need to know about and how they relate to the overall care of your patients.

Medication Reconciliation

As a first responder, you will enter hundreds of homes over your career and find all kinds of medications from all around the world—including homemade remedies from the Far East and homegrown marijuana—that treat a variety of illnesses. What is your responsibility to your patients and the receiving hospital in regard to medication reconciliation?

As paramedics, we tend to work in short spurts, and generally our patient contact time is less than sixty minutes at the time. However, as we leave the emergency department, your patient will be interviewed by many professionals, get tested for a variety of vital markers, and be admitted if necessary. All too often, none of us, including the ED or admitting attending physician, spend enough time reconciling our patients' medications, which could be telltale in their symptomology in regard to overdosing, underdosing, or the synergistic effects of multiple medications.

As paramedics, we also need to respect the cost of medications when they are lost. Many of our elderly patients live from social security check to social security check and can ill afford to purchase additional medication due to misplacement.

It is your role as a *Positude* Paramedic to document *all* medications (including dosages) on your prehospital report or to bring a medication list from your patient to the hospital.

In your work as a *Positude* Paramedic, you are always on the lookout for teaching points. Educating your patients to prepare themselves for a potential medical emergency can save vital minutes in the process of treating them. Be proactive on the minor calls to prepare your patients for the eventual critical call where the minutes will count.

Drug Calculations

Were you a math wizard in high school? If yes, you will likely do well, but if you are one of the many to whom math didn't come easy, you will need to work hard to get through your program and seek tutoring along the way to pass your exams and reach that goal of becoming a paramedic.

This short-term solution is great for passing an exam, but how is this going to work in the middle of nowhere with a patient who is in cardiogenic shock and needs a dopamine drip?

However you learn to manage drug calculations—from mixing medications to drawing up 5 mg of Lopressor—you need to develop a reliable adjunct to set yourself up for success. If you are going to rely on your memory in a time of stress, you are setting yourself up for failure.

As time progresses, we are becoming more and more reliant on technology, which in turn is often dependent on batteries or cellular and Wi-Fi connections. Since there are no guarantees in life, especially when "Murphy" is around, prepare yourself for that moment when you are all on your own, disconnected from the world, and with a life in the balance.

Develop written algorithms, descriptions, and step-by-step instructions to selecting, mixing, drawing up, and administering the right medication at the right time. These instructions should be glued to your equipment in a highly visual location and preferably as close to the medication you need to manage as possible.

As a *Positude* Paramedic, understand your weaknesses and be proactive in your preparation to respond. Don't delay; do it today—if you don't, it's likely it will never get done.

Medication Resource Management

You should never feel alone, regardless of your location, but, as stated above, be prepared to be alone. As technology improves every day, you will have all the information you will ever need at your fingertips. Sometimes we have too many resources and too many opinions; therefore, it is important you take the time to manage your available resources.

I'm not going to endorse or advise which site or app is better or best, but instead I encourage you take some time to research this topic to a greater extent.

Similar to my previous advice, trying to find information or websites to retrieve vital information should not be done at the time of the emergency. Be proactive and line up a separate page on your smartphone with resources including but not limited to:

- Local EMS protocols
- ACLS guidelines
- PALS guidelines
- PHTLS guidelines
- WebMD
- JEMS
- EMS World
- PDR

Part III:

Special Contributors

Before we transition to the one hundred experiences, I have asked a few of my friends to tell you about their past journeys and experiences in health care. Each of them started as a volunteer in their local youth corps and soon thereafter committed their professional lives to emergency services. Each of them has taken a slightly different track along the way and excelled in their respective roles. I hope that you will learn from their stories and see them as options in your own future endeavors.

I close this section with a survivor story and part of the reason I still feel passionate about working as a paramedic today. Each of you will be part of such a story along the way; however, it is rare that you will get an annual thank-you note from a grateful mom, including an update on how your patient is making the most out of the opportunity and second chance in life.

Enjoy!

10

Medical Direction and EMS

Jeffrey S. Rabrich, DO, FACEP, EMT-P

The role of the physician in emergency medical services has evolved quite a bit over the past fifty years as both EMS and technology have evolved and improved. We will explore the role of the physician as it pertains to your daily work as a paramedic in an EMS system, and while no two systems are alike, the principles of EMS medical direction are similar. When you begin a career as a paramedic, you may have little understanding of the role of the physician in your work treating and transporting patients or in how you can develop and improve your relationships and interactions with the physicians you will deal with. Having worked both sides of this relationship over the years in my career, I will discuss what I think are the key strategies for maximizing your interactions with medical control physicians as well as reviewing the elements of physician medical direction (formerly referred to as medical control).

When EMS services first began in the early 1970s, there was no actual requirement to have a physician medical director or even any formal physician involvement with EMS, even though some services did have early physician involvement. Additionally, while EMS was rapidly evolving in the early years, emergency medicine was also becoming a specialty. In fact, it was not recognized as a specialty by the American Board of Medical Specialties until 1979, and as such many of the physicians involved with the early EMS services were not trained in emergency medicine. In reality, several were cardiologists since the early ALS system focused on cardiac care, which included defibrillation and cardiac medications. Some of the very early systems even required a physician or ICU nurse to be present on the ambulance for the paramedics to even practice their skills. We have certainly come a long way from those early years—now paramedics and advanced emergency medical technicians (AEMTs) are able to perform a vast number of skills not only without a physician present but without even making direct contact with a physician. The field of EMS medicine has changed dramatically as well, with EMS now recognized as a board-certified subspecialty. As such, EMS physicians possess a much greater skill level in EMS and a greater understanding of the role of the EMS providers at all levels of training.

The EMS Medical Director

While the laws and regulations vary from state to state, virtually all agencies that provide advanced life support–level care as well as most basic life-support agencies are required to have a physician medical director. The medical director has many roles within the organization and should be actively involved with the providers working for the agency. The agency medical director in most cases will be a different individual from the physicians, providing online medical direction. The medical director sets the medical standards for an agency such as training requirements, continuing medical education (CME), and the medical operating standards for an agency; the director also provides expert medical opinion and case review/quality standards. Depending on where you practice, your agency medical director may be responsible for writing and approving treatment protocols or the director may participate on a larger committee that sets protocols for a region or state such as a regional emergency medical advisory committee (REMAC) or a state emergency medical advisory committee (SEMAC).

It is extremely important to cultivate a good relationship with your medical director as this can lead to improved knowledge and skill as a provider, valuable guidance and sharing of current medical knowledge, advancement within your agency, and overall improved job satisfaction for you, the field provider. Now that EMS is a subspecialty of emergency medicine, most agency medical directors (especially in large agencies) are emergency physicians, and many are now EMS-certified physicians and have completed EMS fellowships or worked as EMS providers themselves.

Offline Medical Direction

Multiple forms of medical direction are given to the EMS providers to enable them to administer prehospital care. Offline medical direction is the written guidance provided to the advanced provider that is not specific to any individual patient but provides guidance on how to treat a variety of conditions. This direction is in the form of written protocols and policy agreed upon by the committee or individuals responsible for writing protocols, and it is approved by any required regulatory agencies. This is the form of medical direction that provides the steps the EMS provider may carry out without speaking with a physician. These tasks are referred to as *standing orders* and are actually equivalent to a physician order for a specific patient and thus issued as a "standing order." The number of steps that can be completed as standing orders vary by both individual protocol and region or state. The remaining steps are listed as "medical control" options, meaning these steps can only be completed in consultation with a physician through "online" medical direction. The reason I am mentioning offline direction and written protocols is to emphasize that these are not set in stone; they will need to change and evolve over time as both EMS capabilities and medicine progress. I work in the New York City EMS system, and fairly regularly I am approached by paramedics from both my own and other agencies who ask good, well-informed questions about why certain protocols are written the way they are or why a particular step is not a standing order. The field providers, in my opinion, have a responsibility to question protocols or procedures that they feel impede care or could be improved. Get involved with your medical director or your REMAC. In other words, as Gandhi said, "Be the change you want to see in the world."

Online Medical Direction

The online medical direction provided during an EMS call can be a chore and source of frustration or a productive and satisfying experience depending on how it's approached and, in some cases, who you are speaking with. Just like EMS and medicine, the contact with online medical direction has evolved in both technical quality and content. In the early days, communication was accomplished through UHF radio and the transmission of a rhythm strip or vital signs over a radio referred to as *telemetry*. In New York City, the centralized facility is still referred to as telemetry even though we don't transmit telemetry data by radio any longer. Some people erroneously refer to this process as medical control, and I've even heard some nurses and physicians answer the phone as "medical control." The term *medical direction* is preferable as the function of this process is for the physician to provide medical direction to the crew with regard to treating that particular patient. It is not a process for "controlling" the paramedics, and thus the name "medical control" has a fairly negative connotation.

So how do you make "the call" go well? You have worked or will work with a partner who claims, "I always get orders from medical control." If so, listen carefully to how these people present themselves on the phone, as you will see some patterns. We have all heard the phrase "a picture is worth a thousand words," and since the physician on the other end of the phone cannot see the patient, basically you need to paint a picture of that patient's condition in way less than a thousand words. The call can be thought of as having distinct parts: the opening, the body, the "ask," and the closing. In some regions, you may be speaking to a central medical direction facility that has a physician solely dedicated to this task; however, this is not the norm. Most often you will be calling the facility that you will be transporting the patient to or another emergency department, and the physician will be seeing patients and will need to be "pulled away" to come to the phone and speak with you. You as the paramedic must keep this fact in mind and realize that you will only be getting a brief moment of the physician's undivided attention, and because of this, you must be clear and concise. The opening of the call is important. Once you introduce yourself, set the stage by saying up front what you think is going on. For example, "Doc, this is Medic XYZ, and I have a fifty-two-year-old male with anaphylaxis to nuts," or "I have a twenty-two-year-old female in status asthmaticus." Why do this? It paints a picture immediately since we have all seen patients with these conditions. If I were the doctor, I would now be listening to everything that comes next in the conversation in the context of the patient having that condition as opposed to wondering where is the medic was going with this.

Next is the body of the call, or when you need to present your case, and it can't be emphasized enough that if you neglect to follow the standard medical format you will lose your audience. A case should be presented beginning with the history of the presenting illness or the story of what's going on. Keep this relevant by only including pertinent positives or negatives. The physician doesn't care that the patient's last meal was at 6:00 p.m. and it was Chinese food, unless it's relevant to the case. Next, after mentioning any past medical or social history that is important to the current problem, a brief summary of your findings from the physical exam should follow. Again, this should be a problem-focused exam, so for the asthmatic patient you need to discuss lung sounds, but her skin turgor to extremity exam probably isn't relevant. Finally, conclude with your assessment of what you think is going on and what you have done up to this point, and then ask for any medical control options you think are needed. A good paramedic should be able to present all this information in sixty to ninety seconds on the phone. Anything that is longer or more drawn out runs the risk of losing the attention of the physician on the phone who may have to get back to other patients. Some paramedics will present their findings and then just wait for the physician to ask questions, say something, or maybe tell them what to do. I always advise my EMS providers that if they think a patient needs a treatment that is a medical control option, then they should ask for it.

After the Call

It is important to continue cultivating the relationship with the physicians you will work with and receive medical direction from. A good way to do this is through follow-up. When you return to that same facility later in your shift, ask how your patient did or what was found, or maybe you could even ask if the doctor has a minute to show you any imaging that may be interesting to the case. This demonstrates that as physicians you are interested in your patient's outcome, the medicine involved, and your continued learning, and, besides, most of us, like to teach. Additionally, if you've recently read about a new treatment or an interesting article about treatment, ask about it and have a discussion. As physicians providing medical direction, we are much more likely to trust and give orders to the paramedic who presents a case well and shows an interest.

In summary, the relationship between the provider and the physician (or an advanced practice provider or nurse if your system allows them to provide medical direction) is the key to both excellent patient care and improved job satisfaction for the EMS provider. Don't be afraid to ask, "Hey, Doc, is there anything I could have done differently or better on that call?"

About the Contributor:

Dr. Jeffrey Rabrich has been involved in EMS for over twenty-five years. Dr. Rabrich started his career in EMS as a volunteer EMT in Rockland County, New York, and has worked as an EMT, paramedic, and flight medic. Dr. Rabrich has worked as a field paramedic in the NYC EMS system as well as Rockland County, New York. Dr. Rabrich is a graduate of the New York College of Osteopathic Medicine, and he completed a residency in emergency medicine at Saint Luke's–Roosevelt Hospital in Manhattan, where he served as chief resident. After residency, Dr. Rabrich served as the EMS medical director at Saint Luke's–Roosevelt Hospital until 2012, and he is currently the medical director of the emergency department at Mount Sinai Saint Luke's Hospital and the vice-chair of the NYC REMAC. He has authored several book chapters on EMS and emergency medicine and is a lead editor of the textbook *Critical Care Transport*.

11

Medical Legal Consideration: So Help Me God?

Joel Hirshfield, Esq., EMTP

"I swear to tell the truth, the whole truth, and nothing but the truth, so help me God (although you may affirm)." Tachycardia, chest tightening, agitation, and difficulty concentrating—you have treated many patients with this presentation of symptoms, but right now this is how you feel as you take your seat on the witness stand. You never expected to be in this situation, but now you are nervous and hoping your actions were proper and "legally" substantiated.

Legal considerations are a relentless presence in all aspects of health care. One way for caregivers to reduce their level of fear about being involved in a legal action is to give diligent attention to the various elements that contribute to the quality of care they provide: skills maintenance, continuing education, protocol familiarity and compliance, proper documentation, and interpersonal communications with nurses; doctors; and, most importantly, patients and their families. Both you and your partner are equally responsible for everything that is done with the patient. Always make sure to look out for each other!

However, the concern of any profession—especially professions related to health care—is that the potential for litigation looms over each decision. The field of emergency care, no matter what the setting, is predominantly governed by civil law, which places legal, ethical, and moral responsibilities on the crew. The categories of law include criminal and civil law, with tort law being the chief civil concern for all prehospital care. Prehospital emergency care providers can be sued by anyone, even if they perform appropriately. However, the burden of proof is on the person bringing the lawsuit (the plaintiff).

One of the areas of greatest concern for us is the gray area of RMAs, or refusing medical assistance. The right to refuse treatment, a basic right of all patients, is based on a fundamental concept that every person of adult age and sound mind has a right to determine what is done or not done to his or her body. Providing care without this consent puts you at risk of liability for assault or battery, even if the care is necessary to save the patient's life.

If the patient refuses care, you must explain the possible consequences and make certain to create thorough and concise documentation. Patients who refuse treatment may be afraid or in emotional distress. Attempting to calm them with rational explanations and reassurance may lead to them consenting. If a patient persists in refusing treatment, follow local protocol, which will most likely include contacting medical control. Even if it doesn't, if there is any concern at all, it is always good practice to utilize and contact medical control and document the interaction with the physician.

To minimize legal risk, explain to the patient what may be wrong, the treatment that is indicated and why, and the consequences that may result without the treatment. Urge the patient to obtain medical care with a personal physician. When possible, encourage a family member to stay with the patient until the patient agrees to seek care or the condition resolves. Attempt to obtain signatures on the EMS record from the patient and witnesses, verifying that the patient is refusing care or transport. Keep in mind that you and your partner are **not** witnesses. Thorough documentation should include the patient's history, your physical findings (including indications of the patient's mental competence), the stated reasons for refusing treatment, and any explanations or advice you have given to the patient or family members. It is very important to clearly and concisely document everything.

Special consideration must be given to patients who may be impaired by the influence of alcohol or drugs, those who may exhibit suicidal tendencies, those who may have signs of a head injury, or those who are not behaving normally according to family members—patients in these cases may not be competent enough to make rational decisions. In these situations, seek assistance from the police and obtain online medical direction. In general, restraint and transport against a patient's will constitute a rare circumstance that could occur after a patient has been determined incompetent to make health-care decisions. Never, ever forget to document all of this!

In *Lemann v. Essen Lane Daiquiris, Inc.*, paramedics were called to a bar by police officers to evaluate an intoxicated man for a hand injury. When they arrived there, they found Parker Lemann. Mr. Lemann was able to answer the paramedics' questions and told them that "he got into a fight, punched someone, and his hand was hurting." The paramedics found that he was alert, and Mr. Lemann told them that he had no other complaints. His vital signs were all normal. His pupils were equal and reactive to light.

The paramedics at the scene offered to take Mr. Lemann to the hospital twice, and both times he refused to go to the hospital. Mr. Lemann then signed a form acknowledging his refusal of transport. Police officers took Mr. Lemann home, but several hours later he was found unconscious by neighbors. He was then transported to a hospital and diagnosed with a fractured skull and a subdural hematoma. He died two days later. Mr. Lemann's parents filed a lawsuit against the paramedics and their employer. They argued that paramedics should have taken Mr. Lemann to the hospital in spite of his lack of consent to be transported. The court found that paramedics were not required to take Mr. Lemann to the hospital because he had the right to refuse transportation. The court further found that "the EMS personnel must balance fulfilling a person's emergency medical needs with respecting a person's wish not to be treated or transported to the hospital." The court found that in this case paramedics were not aware of Mr. Lemann's head injury, and therefore they were proper in respecting his refusal of transport to the hospital. The court granted judgment for the paramedics. This was only possible because of the thoroughness of the paramedics and their complete and legible documentation.[1]

Another more recent but also exceptionally significant concern is the notorious Health Insurance Portability and Accountability Act of 1996 (a.k.a. HIPAA). As health-care workers, we see and hear confidential information every day on the job. We get so accustomed to being around this kind of information that it's easy to forget how important it is to keep it private. Privacy and confidentiality are basic rights in our society. Safeguarding that right is our ethical and legal obligation—HIPAA was enacted to protect just that.

The patient has a right to expect that any information obtained in preparation for, during, or after transport will be kept confidential. Legal protection for this expectation was given with the implementation of HIPAA in 1996. The Privacy Rule portion of HIPAA obligates health-care personnel to ensure that confidentiality of patient information is maintained.

There are potential legal consequences for violating HIPAA, including civil penalties (fines) of up to $250,000, criminal penalties, and personal liability. The Privacy Rule protects the confidentiality of protected health information (PHI). PHI includes individually identifiable information (such as name, Social Security number, and date of birth), health information (such as laboratory results and medical history), and demographic information (such as address and telephone number). It is important to note that HIPAA protects PHI in *any* form, whether it is written, verbal, or electronic. A criminal violation occurs when a provider knowingly discloses PHI for a purpose not permitted under HIPAA and with the intent to use the PHI for personal gain. Note the "knowingly" standard for criminal prosecutions. This means that inadvertent disclosure will not bring criminal sanctions; however, civil sanctions may still result.

In *Pachowitz v. LeDoux*, in 2003, four EMS personnel, including volunteer EMT Katherina LeDoux, responded to a 911 call at the Pachowitz residence for a possible overdose. Approximately two weeks earlier, LeDoux had learned from her friend, Sally Slocomb, that Pachowitz, a work colleague, had a medical condition. After the emergency call, LeDoux, believing that Slocomb and Pachowitz were close friends, spoke to Slocomb about having transported Pachowitz. LeDoux testified that she called Slocomb because she was concerned about Pachowitz and thought Slocomb could help Pachowitz. Slocomb then drove to West Allis Memorial Hospital, where she and Pachowitz worked. There, she discussed Pachowitz's emergency call with staff. Pachowitz later filed suit against LeDoux and won![2]

Finally, though not any less important in any way, all health-care personnel are taught the importance of documentation. Accurate and complete documentation is never more important than when dealing with a patient who is seriously ill or in critical condition. When a patient's status changes rapidly and without warning, numerous interventions are carried out. It is often a challenge to keep up with documentation during a call that requires you to keep constant attention on the patient.

Good documentation serves as protection for EMS personnel, and a complete and accurate report is a reflection of **good patient care**. An accurate, complete, legible medical record implies accurate, complete, organized assessment and management. Include all requested information. If information requested does not apply, note "not applicable" or "N/A." Failure to document implies failure to consider. If you look for something and it is not there, document its absence. **If it is not documented, it was not done.**

The documentation must be legible. If you cannot read the report, you may be unable to determine what happened. Documents presented in court must "speak for themselves." If a document cannot be deciphered, the jury has the right to ignore it altogether. If spaces are provided for documenting times, fill them in carefully. Failing to document times implies lack of concern about the time factor, which is one of the most basic aspects of a call. Although you may be writing the report, your partner or crew has just as much responsibility to make sure it is accurate and should be involved in the writing of the report.

If the report is sloppy, others will assume that the care was equally sloppy. The implementation of electronic medical records (EMRs) and the use of tablets eliminate sloppiness as a factor, but that does not excuse the need for accuracy and completeness. Although legibility is not a factor with tablets, significant care must be taken that the form is not automatically filled based on "check boxes." Every patient is unique, and the final report must be reviewed completely. It is essential that a completed run report paints an accurate and detailed picture of everything that occurred. **Good documentation is a reflection of good patient care!** You must keep in mind that you may be asked to defend yourself in a court of law, and your documentation has to be your best friend, not your enemy!

Most importantly, **never** forget that the patient is a person with feelings and concerns. The same is true for the patient's family or friends. They are also people. You want everyone to be comfortable and secure in your care, and the best way to do that is to get them to trust you and to like you! The first line of protection against legal problems lies in maintaining a professional and compassionate demeanor. Treat patients, family members, and personnel at the facilities with respect, and cooperate fully with other agencies to ensure continuity of care. Make it clear that you care about the patient's well-being and are doing everything possible to serve it. This is why you went to school to become an emergency care provider. Everything that is done from the time the tones drop until the patient is properly transferred to hospital personnel must be focused on your patient and how that patient is affected.

Thorough, concise, and legible documentation, as well as an appropriate concerned compassionate approach to each and every patient, will never do you wrong. If this is accomplished, then you should never have to worry about a knock at the door and being handed a subpoena, "so help you God!"

Notes

1. Lemann v. Essen Lane Daiquiris, Inc., 923 So. 2d 627 (2006).

2. Pachowitz v. LeDoux, 2003 WL 21221823 (Wis. App., May 28, 2003).

About the Contributor:

Joel became an EMT and EMS volunteer in Rockland County in 1979. He became a paramedic in 1980 and began working in the Yonkers 911 system in 1980 for A-A Ambulance and then Empress Ambulance.

He migrated to New York City and worked midnights in the NYC EMS 911 system in Midtown Manhattan. During that time, he assisted in bringing paramedics to Rockland County by becoming one of the original paramedics in North Rockland for Nyack Hospital and serving as a volunteer paramedic for the South Orangetown Volunteer Ambulance Corps. He has continued to care for the people of Rockland County and currently has been with Rockland Paramedic Services for over thirty years.

Joel has also been a practicing trial attorney for over twenty-two years. He is admitted to practice in and before the courts of the state of New York, the Supreme Court of the United States of America, and the federal district courts of the Southern District of New York and the Eastern District of New York. Joel is a member of the American Bar Association, the New York State Bar Association, the New York County Lawyers' Association, and the Westchester County Bar Association, as well as the Association of Trial Lawyers of America and New York City Trial Lawyers Association. Hirshfield & Costanzo, P.C., is a trial litigation firm that also serves as general counsel for volunteer ambulance corps, supporting them and their members in dealing with their everyday legal obligations and interactions.

12

From EMT to MD

Sean Kivlehan, MD

I like to say that as I climbed the ladder I took the time to enjoy every rung. As an attending emergency medicine physician, being a junior ambulance volunteer sometimes feels like a lifetime ago. In many ways, it was. That is how my health-care experience began, at the age of thirteen. Over the next twenty years, I would work as an EMT and paramedic, teach the courses and write the textbooks, and go on to college and medical school, receive a master's degree in public health, finish my residency and fellowship, and become a full-fledged emergency physician. Despite these many years of formal education, it is my paramedic training and experience that I fall back on every single day at work.

These days, when I care for a patient, I am just one member of a much larger team that includes residents, physician assistants, nurses, EMS, various technical assistants, registration staff, security, janitors, administrators, and specialist consultants. On the ambulance, my partner and I filled all of these roles on every call. In fact, we filled even more roles on top of that as lifters and carriers of people and ambulance drivers. When you look at it this way, it isn't surprising that being a paramedic is the best preparation possible for a physician.

Paramedics have tremendous autonomy, making critical decisions with limited information, and they are frequently subjected to intense retrospective review by those who weren't there. You develop a sharp instinct for sick versus not sick as a paramedic, along with an extra-thick skin. If you don't, you won't last long in the field. It is a job that is unique in its simultaneous mental and physical demands: after running a megacode in a hot apartment, you then get to carry that patient down a few flights of stairs. In the field, you are doing everything with only two people until backup arrives—if it is available. Compare this to the team I am a part of in the ED, and you can see why even my hardest days now pale in comparison to a rough shift on "the bus."

The blood and sweat a paramedic sheds to perfect the craft is not for waste. It is what makes the profession what it is: a team, a family really, of extremely well-trained health-care professionals who will respond to any problem, anywhere, anytime. They form the safety net of our society, and like the ED, are the option of last resort for many. Even more, being a paramedic provides the perfect foundation to build upon with further education.

In the ED, I can easily become removed from the patient by a few degrees by the many layers of help, but when things get hairy, I'm expected to step in and fix things. Being a paramedic gave me the framework I needed to confidently manage any crashing patient with a calm authority. Medical school and residency added the components, but it will always be the paramedic in me that saves lives when it matters most. Except now, I don't have to restock and clean the ambulance afterward.

About the Contributor:

Sean Kivlehan, MD, MPH, is an attending physician in the emergency department at the Brigham and Women's Hospital in Boston, Massachusetts. He is the associate director of the International Emergency Medicine Fellowship, a faculty member at Harvard Medical School, and an affiliated faculty member at the Harvard Humanitarian Initiative. He was a paramedic for ten years in New York City and nearby Rockland County, and before that he was an EMT, dispatcher, and junior ambulance volunteer. He trained EMTs and paramedics in many of the New York City area programs and still writes for a number of EMS publications and textbooks.

13

So You Want to Be a Wilderness Paramedic

Frank DiGianni, NREMTP

Excited, frantic, and out of breath, the young hiker showed up at the Beaver Meadows Ranger Station in Rocky Mountain National Park, claiming his father had fallen off Hallett Peak while attempting to climb it. He further stated that his father was badly injured, and although he was still conscious and alert when he left his father to get help, that was more than three hours ago. He gave his father's location, which was at the base of the northeast face of Hallett Peak; he was lying in the snow midway up Tyndall Glacier.

Immediately several rangers were notified: myself, a law enforcement ranger and wilderness paramedic, and John Gillette, a backcountry mountaineering ranger and EMT. The report had been dispatched just after 6:00 p.m. on a Friday, and John and I were the only rangers available at the time. John and I then met up at the ranger station within twenty minutes to load up equipment and formulate a rescue plan. We considered a helicopter rescue, but high winds and fierce snow squalls up on the mountains made that too dangerous. Our next option, and really the only one available, would be to hike up there and locate the fallen climber.

It was now close to 7:00 p.m.; it was mid-August with only about an hour of navigable daylight left. Tyndall Glacier is located approximately five miles up the Flattop Mountain Trail; it is not a true glacier but rather a permanent snowfield that over eons had formed on the saddle between Hallett Peak and Flattop Mountain. The trail begins at the Bear Lake trailhead and is an endless series of switchbacks that goes straight up and over the mountain. In order to access the victim, there would be 3,500 feet of elevation gain up and around Flattop Mountain, and then about a 750-foot elevation drop to the injured man's location midway down the glacier.

By the time John and I reached the trailhead at the end of Bear Lake Road, some ten miles from the ranger station, it was nearing 7:30 p.m., and daylight was fading fast. John carried mostly rescue gear, sleeping bags, ropes, ice axes, slings, carabineers, and an emergency shelter. I carried mostly medical gear, which consisted of trauma dressings and duct tape, collapsible traction splints, cervical collars, and more duct tape; ten 1,000 cc bags of IV fluid as well as pain medications; a Laerdal handheld suction device; intubation equipment; a bag-valve mask (BVM); and Mylar blankets...lots of Mylar blankets. We each carried approximately twenty-five to thirty pounds of gear, plus enough water and food to last at least the next twenty-four hours.

It was a long, arduous grunt up the dimly lit and very steep trail. It was well maintained but also well worn since it is a popular hiking trail. But hiking the trail at night was discouraged and could be very treacherous; you could easily plunge hundreds if not thousands of feet to your death with one false step. Hiking with bulky packs and headlamps made the going cautious and slow. By the time John and I reached the top of the glacier, it was after 10:00 p.m., and although the temperature at the forested trailhead had been pleasant, the glacier was 1,500 feet above tree line and exposed to the elements, sitting at almost thirteen thousand feet above sea level. Temperatures on the glacier were well below freezing, and there was a constant biting wind that was inescapable.

Using ice axes and crampons, we could make our way down the glacier to the location of the victim in another hour. At this point he had been injured at least eight or nine hours earlier, and John and I both assumed we would find a frozen body and that it would turn into a recovery operation. But to our amazement, we found the victim, a German tourist named Thorstein, quite alive but also in dire need of emergency medical treatment.

In a thick German accent, the victim explained that he had slid almost two hundred feet down the face of the mountain. Although he had a minor head wound, he remembered the incident and had never lost consciousness, but now he was hypothermic and very lethargic. His injuries consisted of severely bruised ribs, a possibly fractured pelvis, and a definitely fractured femur. He also had numerous minor injuries, but none of those had appeared to be life threatening.

Thorstein's biggest life threat at the moment was the cold: his oral temperature, as indicated by a digital thermometer, was ninety-four degrees. We had to get him out of the elements and into a shelter. He was wearing mostly Gore-Tex and fleece, which had kept him dry, but lying on the icy snowfield for so many hours had robbed him of his body heat.

John and I erected the emergency shelter, which was really nothing more than a small domed tent, and carefully we dragged Thorstein inside. I placed hot packs inside his fleece undergarments and under his armpits and groin too, and I wrapped him in Mylar blankets and a sleeping bag. Using a camp stove and a pot of melted snow, I began heating 1,000 cc bags of normal saline. The stove also served to provide some heat inside the shelter.

I established two IVs, one in each arm, and when the saline was about one hundred degrees, I began to infuse the warm fluids as rapidly as possible. After about an hour, Thorstein's oral temp was now 95.5 degrees and he was more alert. With the threat of hypothermia diminishing, it was now time to further assess him and address his injuries.

He had a carotid pulse of about 50 bpm, and I wasn't able to get a blood-pressure reading. He had shallow respirations with fine basilar rales, a possible sign of high-altitude sickness. His pelvis was tender and slightly unstable but his abdomen was soft, so I didn't suspect any major internal bleeding. His left femur was slightly angulated and his left foot pointing inward; it appeared as if he had two knees. He had no distal pulse, but in fairness he had no other distal pulses either, most likely from hypothermia and not from hypovolemia.

I directed John to stabilize above and below the fracture while I applied manual traction to straighten out the abnormal extremity; Thorstein screamed out from the excruciating pain. Then, using duct tape, I secured his left leg to his right. I also duct-taped his pelvis, which provided alleviation of the tenderness and gave it stability. It was now approaching 2:00 a.m. John went out to cut steps into the snowfield up to the trail in order to make extrication a little easier, while I continued to monitor and treat Thorstein.

While John and I were doing our respective tasks, back at the ranger station efforts were underway to put together an extraction team. A squad of ten to twelve rangers would hike up to our location at first light to retrieve Thorstein and get him back down to the trailhead. They would be packing ropes, technical rescue gear, blankets, oxygen, a backboard, a Stokes litter, and a specialized gurney with one big wheel under the center that is sometimes referred to as "The Mule."

The night was bitterly cold, and three inches of fresh snow had fallen, and the constant flapping of the shelter walls under the strong winds coming down the mountain was deafening. I stayed awake, changing Thorstein's IV bags often while he had restless on-and-off sleep. With as much fluid as I had pumped into him, he needed to urinate frequently; at first I used a plastic cup, but in order for that to work I had to remove many of his blankets and clothes, which further exposed him to the cold. A Foley catheter would have made things a lot easier, but lacking one I resorted to making one using a latex glove, a 12-French suction catheter, an empty IV bag, and yes...duct tape. In this way I was able to gauge both accurate urinary output and clarity. My patient was as stable and as comfortable as I could make him; all we needed to do now was to wait for the extraction team to arrive.

By 9:30 a.m. the team was making its way down the steps John had sliced into the glacier and heading toward our location. The team leader, Mountaineering Ranger Jim Detterline, had directed his squad to set up a Tyrolean traverse, which uses ropes, pulleys, and anchor points to hoist the Stokes litter and bring it up the glacier. The patient was secured to a backboard with duct tape, wrapped in blankets, and placed into the Stokes litter. Although Thorstein had an uncomfortable night, his oral temperature was just about ninety-seven degrees, and he had diminished pain and strong distal pulses.

By the time the team had hauled Thorstein off the ice and to the Flathead Mountain trail at the top of Tyndall Glacier, another two hours had passed. I stayed with Thorstein the entire time. I had placed a blood-pressure cuff over both IV bags and placed them under the blankets that now cocooned him to prevent the fluids from turning to ice. It took another five and a half hours to make it down the rugged mountainous trail, with the patient being transported in "The Mule" and three to four rangers holding on to each side. At the steeper and more treacherous parts of the trail, ropes were again used to provide a braking system for the litter.

At the trailhead was a waiting transport helicopter, AirLife from Denver General Hospital, as well as Thorstein's anxious son. I transferred the patient care over to the flight crew and said my auf Wiedersehens to my patient. The flight time would be about thirty minutes, and by the time Thorstein arrived at Denver General, it would have been just about twenty-six hours since he had fallen. For about seventeen of those hours I provided direct and constant patient care. After completing my paperwork and a long debriefing session, I was finally able to get some sleep after having been awake and "running" on honey, raisins, and chocolate for nearly forty straight hours.

The aforementioned incident took place on August 16 and 17, 1991, and should be used as an example of what being a paramedic in a remote wilderness area can be like. Unlike their EMT and paramedic counterparts who work in urban or suburban locations where the closest hospital is just a few blocks or a few miles away, wilderness medics face immense challenges presented by the wilderness and remote locations.

As a wilderness medic you must be skilled and competent in technical rope rescue, which includes high-angle rescue and swift water rescue. If you can't gain access to the victim, you are of no use to that victim and could possibly become a victim yourself. It's not enough to just "treat for shock," give oxygen, and pump in IV fluids or pain management medications; you must also take great care in the maintenance of those fluids and medications. Hydration and homeostasis need to be balanced along with nutritional requirements. At some point your patient will need to drink fluids and eat, and he will also need to urinate and defecate— that's your responsibility too.

A wilderness medic must be more than a paramedic: you are also part critical-care nurse, part nurse's aide, part respiratory therapist, and in some cases, such as when reducing dislocations or providing field amputations, you must also be part physician. Having the improvisation skills of a MacGyver or an Eagle Scout is also helpful. In many wilderness areas paramedics often have greater latitude in standing orders and treatment modalities and function with limited or no direct medical control, and you could potentially be caring for your patient for as long as several hours to several days. Arduous extrications in remote isolated locations, exacerbated by the long-term patient care aspect, are what make wilderness medicine unique among all other forms of EMS.

Although I was originally trained as a paramedic in New York City, I sought out the training and certification required to be a wilderness paramedic on my own, often at my own expense. Courses such as Wilderness EMT Training, Wilderness Survival Training, Search and Rescue Training, High and Low Angle Technical Rope Rescue, Swift Water Rescue, and Orienteering (which is the ability to navigate using a topographical map and compass) all helped to prepare me for the rigors of functioning as a wilderness medic. For seven years of my career, from 1988 until 1994, the National Park Service provided me the opportunity to utilize those skills, and I did it in some of the most scenic but accessibly isolated places in the country.

The scenery and the wildlife were spectacular, but the compensation was low and the working conditions were often intolerable. As they say in National Park Service circles, "Rangers take their pay in sunsets." But it was the enormous responsibilities due to the very nature of the job that fulfilled me, plus it provided me with life experience and personal gain and rewards that have yet to be equaled...and I say this as I approach my fortieth year of employment in all forms of EMS. As a United States National Park Ranger and wilderness caregiver, I never had it so good while simultaneously having it so bad.

About the Contributor:

Native New Yorker Frank DiGianni was born in 1955 in the Bronx and was raised in the northern suburbs. He is a graduate of Alfred State College of New York, Saint Vincent's Institute of Emergency Medicine, New York City, New York, where he earned his Paramedic Certification, and also a graduate of The National Ranger Training Academy, Nelsonville, Ohio, where he received his Federal Law Enforcement training.

In a career that began in 1977, he has been a New York State Park ranger, a United States National Park ranger, a marine patrol officer, a paramedic, a flight medic, a paramedic instructor, a high-angle rescue instructor, a constable, and a wildlife rehabilitator.

He has traveled to all fifty states and to forty-four countries and has been on wilderness expeditions that have taken him to all seven continents.

He resides with his wife, Kim, and three dogs in the Catskill Mountains of southern New York State.

14

A Woman's Perspective

Lieutenant Bernadette Frae, BS, EMT-Paramedic

I thought that growing up with five sisters had prepared me for life. It made me tough but caring, strong but gentle—I got lots of tough love, but it taught me to love. I was most grateful for having loving and caring parents who were true role models for life.

My EMS career started some twenty-five years ago in New York City, New York, when at a tender age of sixteen years I was standing in line at the local grocery store when my life changed forever.

Right in front of me, two men started arguing, fists flew, and next thing I witnessed was one of the men crashing through a large plate-glass window.

After the initial shock, I saw blood everywhere and knew I had to do something. I ran to the first-aid aisle to retrieve supplies, grabbed all I could, and rushed back to the patient's side. I applied direct pressure and bandages and waited for the medics to arrive.

After watching my older sister serve for the past eight years in her role as a paramedic, I knew that I wanted to do something in the field of medicine but just didn't quite know what it would be.

Fast-forward five years: I joined the local volunteer ambulance corps and immediately knew this was my calling as well.

Having learned from my sister's experience, I knew this was a male-dominated profession, and that being recognized as an equal, it would not be a cakewalk.

Throughout my years as a paramedic student and eventually as a full-fledged paramedic, I learned many lessons along the way. I'm extremely proud of my accomplishments and contribution to this profession; however, I find that being a woman in a man's world requires some additional effort to be considered equal or to stay ahead.

The lessons I want to share are these: the importance of knowing who you are and to never lower your personal standards and ethics just for the sake of wanting to belong to the "good old boys' club." If you work harder, study more, and hold your ground when challenged, you will often find yourself being treated the same as the rest. Don't open the door (not even once), don't tolerate inappropriate behavior, and most importantly, resist dating within your chosen profession.

All that I've just mentioned will be major factors, especially early in your career. Once you have established yourself as a true professional who maintains healthy personal boundaries, they will see you as an equal.

Now that I've gotten this off my chest, let's go over the unique challenges of being a woman and a paramedic.

One of the best days of your life will be the day you find out that you are pregnant. The euphoria will wear off soon enough—just as soon as you realize that you are now responsible for more than just yourself. You'll have flashbacks of all the calls where you could have been exposed to microorganisms in less than environmentally sanitary situations or of the times when you were running ten jobs on a hot summer day.

I'm not discouraging you female readers from joining a profession that has given me so much. I just want you to be aware of the challenges that lie ahead. How can you best prepare yourself to be six, seven, or even eight months pregnant and still be staring down an EDPs, working a cardiac arrest, or crawling into a crashed car?

You can do this by understanding your limitations, establishing strong partnerships, and getting your spouse's support.

I carried three pregnancies to full term without any major complications. It wasn't always smooth sailing, but being an alpha mom, I figured out how to change diapers, do laundry, make sandwiches, and get the kids ready for school pictures. I knew my own limitations and decided to live in the now. I learned to dial to the right, meaning that I learned to stop doing the things that were not all that important.

I strongly recommend this gratifying career to my peers with these final instructions: be professional at all times, stay above the fray, and be all that you can be. Don't let anybody determine what your limitations are—work harder, work smarter, and live life to the fullest.

Here's a message with some advice for all paramedics regardless of your gender but from a woman's perspective: Pay attention to the little things when treating your patients. Be mindful of their emergency, be respectful of your surroundings, and never take life for granted.

Be a partner in the mold of someone you admire, be a leader, and lead by example. Arrive on time, be engaged, care for one another, and stay true to yourself.

If I have one wish for all of us, it is that we elevate our profession to the level of a true career, which would allow us to work hard, earn a decent wage, secure our future, and allow us ample time with our families. Don't forget to pay it forward!

About the Contributor:

Native New Yorker Bernadette Frae was born in the New City, New York, and was the youngest of six girls. She is a graduate of Westchester Community College, where she earned her Paramedic Certification. She earned her bachelor degree in Emergency Management from State University of New York.

Her career began in 1995 at Rockland Paramedic Services, and she has been a station lieutenant for the past ten years. She is an active mother of three young children and a small business owner, teaching Advanced Cardiac Life Support to healthcare providers throughout the Hudson Valley region.

15

Responding to a Terrorism-Related Incident:

All-Hazards Approach All the Time

Steven Kanarian, FDNY EMS EMT-Paramedic

Terrorism-awareness training teaches emergency responders that terrorist incidents are more likely to occur during the daytime, on the anniversary of terrorist events, and in government buildings or places of worship. During the month of April, we are all thinking of the Columbine High School massacre and the bombing of the Alfred P. Murrah Federal Building in Oklahoma City. In the post–September 11 world, emergency responders should always have a high degree of suspicion when it involves prominent dates, high-profile locations, and potential secondary events. Safe operations require the use of an all-hazards safety approach to responses involving explosions, multiple patients, and other unusual circumstances.

When responding to a mass-casualty incident (MCI), to prepare for terrorism, there are two main adjustments that need to be made in our response mind-set. The intent of terror organizations is to cause damage and kill civilians and rescuers to gain publicity for their cause. In past years incidents had dangers; in the present world, terrorist incidents are lethal.

Terrorism is different—we are the target.

Trying to identify the cause of a MCI is fruitless. The Oklahoma City Fire Department thought they were responding to a gas explosion on April 19, 1994. The firefighters responding to the World Trade Center in 1993 thought they were responding to a transformer fire. In both the cases, the terrorist origin of the event was not apparent until the smoke cleared and the explosive crater was discovered. In contrast, the airplane flown by Yankees pitcher Cory Lidle that crashed into a Manhattan high-rise in October 2006 was thought to be terrorism but was an accidental crash. When responding to a high-risk incident, we need to follow an all-hazards approach and not depend on determining the cause of the MCI. The safety focus of responding fire companies should be on the hazards while reevaluating the evolving scene for secondary incidents. The best policy is to utilize general safety rules on all responses. By embedding safety procedures in our daily operations, we can develop safety habits that will pay off during a terrorist incident.

Scene Size-Up

Stop. Look. Listen. Think. Allow time for your brain to assess scene hazards and process the information on the scene. The scene assessment begins when we are reviewing the dispatch information. When responding to an incident, it is good safety procedure to have in place a general procedure of stopping at the outermost perimeter of the call location, or when you can first see the building, and watching for key indicators of terrorist incidents. Outward indicators of terrorist incidents such as chemical clouds, dispersal equipment, weapons, gas containers, and other clues may give you forewarning. You know your response area and realize that something looks out of place or deviates from the routine. Stop, look, listen, think, and listen to your instincts.

"Engine 35, Medic 1, respond to Elmwood High School for a difficulty in breathing."

While responding to this call, your dispatcher updates your call information: "Engine 35, Medic 1, you have three patients with shortness of breath and vomiting." Realizing this response is different from the usual asthmatic in the nurse's office, you stop the apparatus as you turn the corner and approach the school. Observation of the scene reveals two police officers coughing and rubbing their eyes and several students with shortness of breath and vomiting. Your scene size-up warns you that this is a potential SLUDGEMS incident (which stands for "salivation, lacrimation, urination, defecation, gastrointestinal upset, emesis, miosis," the symptoms of nerve agent poisoning), requiring isolation suits and decontamination. With a proper scene size-up, we are able to prepare for the appropriate response and not expose members to chemical exposure with inadequate protection. A word of caution: terrorist organizations use an initial event to injure civilians and draw in emergency responders. This tactic was clearly demonstrated in the fictional movie *The Kingdom*, starring Jamie Foxx (I highly recommend this video for use in training sessions or to gain perspective on secondary events). Consideration must be given to clearing the scene of weapons, perpetrators, or explosives prior to initiating search and rescue to reduce the risk of increased injury and deaths from a secondary event. This type of initial response to our school scenario may be a lure for emergency crews into a Columbine-type event with multiple devices.

The magnitude of the Murrah Federal Building, the World Trade Center, and the Madrid train bombing demonstrates an increasing mortality and severity of terrorist incidents. Explosives are the most common weapon used by terrorists to date. Casualty numbers could increase exponentially with the use of chemical and biological weapons. It is important for your team to continually drill plans for implementing rapid decontamination and use of proper protective equipment.

All emergency responders need to improve our knowledge and response methods in expectation of the future. As experienced responders retire, our experience level with terrorism is rapidly dropping. Newer firefighters should be especially diligent in observing the scene size-up, evaluating hazards, suspecting the secondary event, and heeding the lessons learned from previous incidents.

How Do We Prepare for the Unknown?

We can prepare for future incidents by following safety rules on a daily basis and incorporating best practices through training. The most basic safety rule is to use time, distance, and shielding. By minimizing our time exposed to a hazard, maximizing our distance, and using the best shielding available when facing a hazard, we can maximize our safety. When operating at a terror-related event with secondary events, we need to communicate with law enforcement and seek hard cover. *Cover* is protection that can stop bullets and projectiles. Protection behind buildings, concrete walls, and similar obstructions is optimal cover. Standing behind vehicle doors and wood structures is not adequate cover.

Midnight Rules to Live and Stay Alive By

- Stay upwind and upgrade from fumes and liquids.
- Maintain 1,500-foot distance for explosive devices/incidents.
- There should be no radio or cell-phone transmissions at bomb incidents.
- Rule of thumb—if, when holding your thumb up in front of you, you can still see a hazmat incident, you are too close.
- Partially devastated buildings—be aware of secondary bombs.

- Stay two to three times the height of the building away during prolonged fires or buildings damaged from explosions.
- Vary response routes and routine operational tactics.

What Lessons Have We Learned?

In two terrorist incidents, EMS personnel received criticism for rushing to the scene while the terror events were still unfolding. At the Columbine High School massacre, medics were criticized for not waiting for the scene to be determined as safe. During the response to the Columbine massacre, medics entered the school grounds to assist severely injured patients. By entering an active scene of an ultraviolent event in order to rescue injured patients, these paramedics placed themselves in grave danger.

After the Atlanta Olympic Park bombing in 1996, Don Heitt Jr., assistant chief for the Atlanta Fire Department, said, "When medics see patients, they have a tendency to forget the number one rule (safety)."[1] EMS providers were again criticized for engaging patients before the scene had been checked for secondary devices or perpetrators. A secondary device was ignited but did not detonate to full potential. Although these two incidents did not result in injury to emergency responders, the potential for injury or death was present in both events.

A more poignant example of the consequences of terrorist incidents occurred during the response to a chemical weapons attack in the Tokyo subway system, where Sarin was used to attack passengers. During this attack, 135 EMTs (9.4 percent of the total patients from the event) were secondarily exposed to Sarin. In a report on the event, author T. Okamura points out that the Sarin used was only 30 percent strength, and full-strength military

Sarin could have resulted in EMT and paramedic deaths.[2] The symptoms of secondary exposure were alleviated by ventilating ambulances and treatment areas.

What Can We Learn from Other Countries?

The Northern Ireland Fire Department uses tactics to minimize personnel exposure to secondary events:

> "Always handle incidents with the minimum of resources and deploy backups to nearby stations...They have also learned to routinely remove victims to safety and are aware that attacks can include multiple incidents."[3]

The London Fire Brigade, which also deals with terrorism, uses perimeters to control the scene and enforce safety:

> "Two concentric areas are established—the inner cordon and the outer cordon. An outer cordon is established to limit the incident from affecting nearby businesses and homes. An inner cordon is also established to monitor and control crews working at the scene."[4]

This use of perimeters allows the London Fire Brigade control over entering and exiting personnel and promotes accountability. The inner perimeter is used to brief crews about safety concerns before they enter and to debrief them when they exit the inner cordon.

Training

To meet the evolving nature of terrorism, fire departments should be engaged in progressive training that incorporates "out of the box" thinking. What does good training for terrorism look like? Pre-event training should incorporate a scene with multiple hazards and the need to communicate between fire departments, police departments, and EMS. If we train emergency responders to stage and wait for the scene to be cleared of perpetrators and bombs and decontamination setup, we can prevent secondary illness and injury due to unnecessary exposure.

During a terrorist incident, personnel's ability to adapt and solve problems will carry the day. Rescue personnel should seek out as much varied training and knowledge as they can gain access to. Scenarios staged in fire training academies should incorporate hazards requiring police and fire specialty units. Communication between services will save lives in a Columbine-type incident. Frankly, if emergency responders are not trained to stage and wait for a scene to be cleared of explosives, perpetrators, or decontamination setup, they run the risk of large-scale injuries and fatalities to fire department personnel. Scenarios should be staged using real hazards, utilizing children and public servants as patients to challenge responders.

If emergency responders are trained in realistic scenarios with hazards, they will be more likely to survive a terrorist incident in the future. Hard decisions may have to be made, and these ethical/operational issues should be breached in tabletop sessions and drills. We have to train our responders to perform in drills as if they were faced with a real terrorist incident. Emergency responders will only do what they have been trained to perform. Shouldn't we be trained in real situations with multiple hazards while being faced with patients in dire need of care? Now is the time to prepare for the unknown challenges of the future and incorporate lessons learned from past responses.

Action Plan for Terror-Related MCIs:

1.   Stop, look, listen, think
2.   Evaluate limits of PPE
3.   Consider staging until scene is cleared
of explosives and perps.
4.   Reassess for secondary events
5.   Use time, distance, and shielding

Notes

1. M. Nordberg, "Terror at the Olympics," *EMS Magazine* 25, no. 11 (1996): 51–57.

2. T. Okamura, N. Takasu, S. Ishimatsu, S. Miyanoki, A. Mitsuhashi, K. Kumada, et al., "Report on 640 Victims of the Tokyo Subway Sarin Attack," *Annals of Emergency Medicine* 28 (1996): 129–135.

3. G. Buck, *Preparing for Terrorism: An Emergency Services Guide* (Albany: Delmar Publishing, 2002), Page Number/Range.

4. Buck, *Preparing for Terrorism*, Page Number/Range.

City of Oklahoma City, Document Management Team. (1996). Final report, the City of Oklahoma City, Alfred P. Murrah Federal Building Bombing (Stillwater, OK: Fire Protection Publications).

About the Contributor:

Steven Kanarian, MPH, is a retired lieutenant from the New York City Fire Department, EMS Command, who responded to both attacks on the World Trade Center as an urban search and rescue (USAR) medical specialist. Steven has also published *The Downwind Walk*, which is the only book by an EMS professional about 9/11. His website is www.Paramedicmastery.com, and he can be reached on Facebook @Downwindwalk.

16

Family Tragedy: "Survivor Story"

The Riello Family

So this is every parent's worst nightmare!

On December 15, 2007, my husband woke up at 2:00 a.m. Our younger son wasn't home yet; we had let him use the car, and he said he would be home early. But he was still not home, leaving us restless.

I remember my husband being so angry and saying he hated the weekends, and I agreed with him.

That being said, we tossed, turned, and paced the floor, waiting for our younger son to come home, never worrying about Christopher, who was twenty-one and out with friends we knew. We really weren't worried.

That all changed at about 4:30 a.m. when my husband looked out the window and saw a NYS trooper pull into the driveway. It took my breath away; I wondered what happened, immediately thinking the worst. We hurried down to the front door, meeting two NYS troopers standing there with somber faces, hoping for the best but fearing the worst. Neither of my boys was with them.

My nightmare was about to come true: Which of my boys wouldn't be coming home? As I opened the door, I saw the troopers averting their eyes from mine as they asked if we were the parents of Christopher. I had fleeting thoughts of death and mayhem, but not of Chris; he was out and about with friends—what possibly could have gone wrong?

After confirming that we were Chris's parents, they informed us with a shaky voice that our son had been hit by a car on the parkway. None of it made any sense to me at that time.

Taking a few seconds to regroup, I could not comprehend what possibly could have happened hours before. I asked the trooper to repeat it one more time to let it all sink in. Chris was not in a car at the time of the accident but had been walking across the parkway in the southbound lane when he was scooped and nearly fatally wounded.

The only good thing in this moment of despair was the fact that our younger son pulled into the driveway, explaining that he had fallen asleep at his friend's house. Now was not the time to let him know how much we had worried about him.

Confused, angry, hurt, and worried about my husband, I provided the troopers with telephone numbers of his friends, who were supposed to have been with him. The thought that they left him all alone that night still angers me today.

Before leaving, the troopers urged us to go to Westchester Medical Center (WMC) as soon as possible, where he had been airlifted with grave injuries.

Not knowing where to start and forever grateful for my very large Italian family, who were gathering as time went on, we made our way to WMC as quickly as possible, hoping to see Chris.

Soon after arrival, we were informed of Chris's injuries and were asked to identify him, which according to them was standing procedure. As a mother, I couldn't comprehend why until I saw Chris for the first time. There were tubes coming out of every orifice; his face was swollen and scratched up beyond recognition. It took me a few seconds to confirm my worst fears, although I was grateful that he was still alive.

Even though it's been nine years, just writing about this, I feel like I'm back in the room, and I can't help but cry. My poor husband was so distraught and crying uncontrollably that he needed to be removed and consoled by his extended family.

I know we got through it because we always believed that he was going to be OK. He had the most amazing, caring doctors and nurses in the world. Christopher's orthopedic surgeon came to see us soon afterward and explained to the extent possible all of the orthopedic injuries that he was going to address during his first of many surgeries to come.

Not knowing if Chris was going to make it through his first night, we asked our family priest, Father Higgins, to provide the anointing of the sick. All of the nurses and doctors actually took a time-out to say a prayer for wisdom, strength, and God's hands to pull Chris through these difficult times.

Father Higgins came to see us after and attempted to appease us by letting us know that it was a dire situation; however, not once, not even for a single minute, did I believe Chris would not pull through.

We waited nearly twelve hours with lots of acts of kindness by both the staff and other family members, and then our vascular surgeon informed us that he was able to restore circulation to Chris's right leg by transplanting veins from his left leg to his nearly amputated right leg.

When we finally saw Chris again, he had three large external fixators in place, which we thought was going to be the worst—until we were told that his main aorta was sheared and leaking, which could essentially cost him his life at any moment.

Seeing him in a critical condition with fluctuating blood pressure, too many drips, and a ventilator, I felt completely overwhelmed and helpless. I gained strength from those around me and especially from the many unnamed heroes who took care of Chris day and night for the months to come.

Thinking back, I got to meet some of the medics and nurses who initially took care of Chris at the scene of the accident, including the civilians and an army staff sergeant who called 911 and kept him alive until the medics arrived.

Every year since Chris's accident, on the anniversary of his accident, I always send out a group Facebook message to what I call "Chris's angels on earth," telling them all how grateful we are that they were all in the right place at the right time to help save Chris's life and that we could never thank them enough! They're all like members of our family!

Christopher was in the trauma unit from December 15, 2007, until January 8, 2008. He had many surgeries during that time to repair his right leg, left femur, aortic tear, fractured right scapula, left upper arm with nerve damage to his hand, left sinus fracture, L1-L2 lumbar fractures, and several significant facial lacerations on his chin, lips, and cheeks.

After his discharge from WMC, it took another six months of hard work at Helen Hayes Hospital before Chris finally made it home, when I took over care by administering IV antibiotics with shaky hands.

I'm forever grateful for God's grace and Chris's angels on earth for giving him a second opportunity at life. Chris has made a near full recovery and has since gone back to school to become an ultrasound technician and is currently in pursuit of his second passion in life—to drive long-haul tractor trailers cross country as soon as he obtains his CDL license.

A grateful mom and dad!

Note from Chris:

I was involved in a terrible accident in 2007, and I was rescued by Walter and his partners on the graveyard shift. I'm forever thankful for them and all the others involved in my rescue. Without them, my second chance at life would not have been possible. I'm grateful for all emergency services personnel, whether paid or volunteers, who sacrifice time with their families. Our medics deal with overwhelmingly stressful situations.

They are the calm in the middle of a raging storm; if it was not for them, I would never have made it to WMC. It was not my time to go, and for this I will be forever grateful.

Part IV: One Hundred Experiences

Over the next one hundred pages, you will get a flavor of what it is like to be a paramedic in different scenarios and circumstances.

Some stories will be serious, some will be sad, while others will have a twisted sense of paramedic humor. Just keep in mind that our devotion to patient care and service excellence is never intentionally compromised.

To protect all involved, names have been omitted on purpose. All stories are told from the writer's perspective, but this does not mean that others could not have seen it differently.

Some of you will likely be medics already. Read these stories and try to relate to the experiences rather than comparing them to your own experiences.

Relate; don't compare.

1

Why I Wanted to Be a Medic

I'm an adrenaline junkie at heart and needed something that would make my heart skip a beat. After careful research and consideration, being a paramedic would fulfill all my needs, or so I thought.

In actuality—all kidding aside—I'd always wanted to be a medical doctor but didn't pay enough attention in school to get grades good enough to propel me into medical school.

It wasn't until I came to the United States that I learned about paramedicine since it was a rather new career option in the early 1990s, especially in Upstate New York.

After I started volunteering with the Hancock Volunteer Rescue Squad and was introduced to the concept of paramedicine by Shawn Kaufman, I was sold. I wanted to be just like Shawn, or so I thought.

Looking back over the past twenty-five years of service, I haven't regretted my decision to become a paramedic, not even once. It has given me everything I've always wanted and that is to make a difference in our patients' lives and to have the opportunity to improve or extend someone's life.

It has been a fun-filled ride full of adrenaline rushes, unexpected situations, sadness, joy, and everything in between.

I **love** being a paramedic!

2

911 Paramedic

If you are an adrenaline junkie and thrive on the unknown, this job is for you. You can have days without a single call or days where the tones never stop going off. Sometimes you will be all by yourself, and other times you will be with an EMT or paramedic partner. You get paid for what you know, not for what you do. It all sounds too good to be true.

Being a 911 medic is still one of the best jobs I have ever had, although I know for sure that not all medics will agree with me, especially those who worked in difficult neighborhoods with many high-rises and few working elevators. I can only imagine how tough this job must be in 115-degree temperatures in downtown Phoenix or in Chicago when it is cold, for example, while working a major vehicle accident (MVA) on an ice-covered road.

What I do know is that being a 911 medic is a great honor; it's a privilege to take care of the sick and injured. It's amazing the people we get to meet, work with, and work for. It's nerve-racking and exciting to treat complex patients in less-than-desirable conditions.

I would not have traded it for the world. So many positive interactions, so many lives affected, changed, and saved. I'm so very lucky to have been—and still be—a 911 paramedic.

Be proud of who you are, and strive to be best at it.

3

The Old Bird Ventilator

Which bird was turned into a ventilator? How do they come up with these silly names?

It really is too bad that most of you will never have the honor to work with the good ole Bird Ventilator—that green transparent boxlike ventilator that none of us really knew how to operate. However, when it started clicking, it did a great job.

The first auto or semiautomatic ventilators were called "humans": paramedics used a bag-valve mask at a rate to sustain life. The Bird Ventilator was a close second and certainly the first mechanical device widely used for emergency critical-care transports.

I truly don't have any great memories of this device other than frustration. I often felt incompetent and reliant on my MacGyver intuition to ensure safe, quality care for my patients.

I can distinctly remember transferring a semiconscious patient on a Bird Ventilator to a NYC hospital in the early 1990s. He was relatively stable and able to communicate using hand signals and eye movement.

After getting settled and en route to NYC, I started experiencing technical difficulties with the Bird Ventilator. After making many adjustments, the patient finally offered to manually bag himself for the remainder of the ride.

It was not the right thing to do; however, it was right for the patient.

4

LP6 Wheel Chock

Who can remember this boat anchor? I remember that when I took it off the table the first time I just about dropped it on the floor. I didn't anticipate the forty pounds of dead weight, and so it just about pulled my arm out of its socket.

Why do I bring this up? We need to reflect on the past at times to appreciate where we came from and how far we have gotten.

Our LP6 was a boxy, heavy, and monophasic EKG/defibrillator with the big paddles—it was meant to be housed in hospital emergency departments, not in back of an ambulance or 911 first-response vehicles.

Fast-forward twenty years, and we have reduced the weight by 50 percent and only use 10 percent of the LP20's capabilities.

Paramedics today have at their fingertips the ability to monitor EKG, SaO_2, CO, CO_2, and MAP as well as obtain a 12-Lead EKG before you wirelessly transmit it to your local cardiac STEMI-receiving center.

It went from a boat anchor with limited capabilities to an advanced machine that gives you more than you can handle.

Before you complain about your current situation, think back to see how far we have come. Next, be part of the upcoming innovation and improvement that will lead to better patient care, experiences, and outcomes.

Be the change you want to see!

5

747 Box

"Boeing 747 ten nautical miles northwest of New York Bravo airspace, requesting vectors for landing at KJFK."

The good ole 747 storage box might as well have been a Boeing 747—it was big and clunky to say the least.

From what I remember going back to 1990, there was not a day we didn't wish we had something more manageable.

Besides being clunky, whenever you opened the box to retrieve supplies, it was inevitable that someone would give it a push or a shove, causing it to tumble and empty its contents all over the floor.

The point of writing this story is not to complain about the past but to encourage you to be creative and cutting edge in giving feedback on the way equipment is designed in order to improve safety and quality of care.

Don't just complain; be part of the solution. Attend trade shows to learn about new advances in your industry. Bring ideas to your bosses with a request to run a trial in your work environment.

Be the change you want to see, or risk being stuck in your Studebaker for life.

6

Transports from Hell

I don't think my paramedic program prepared me to handle a critical-care transport from hell.

I was dispatched to a small hospital in Upstate New York to transport a Level I trauma patient to a trauma center about sixty minutes away. I was instructed to bring my ventilator and as many IV pumps we possessed.

At that time (we are going back a few years), all that we carried were military transport pumps (MTP) and a very basic ventilator.

I remember walking into this very small emergency department's critical-care bay only to see lots of equipment and doctors and nurses scrambling to get this patient ready for transport.

After getting a short report, I tried to collect my thoughts on how I was going to pack six IV pumps, a ventilator, and four chest tubes plus associated equipment in the back of a rather small ambulance.

Stepping back for a minute, I realized that this patient was going to die at the current facility not because of incompetence but because they had done everything they could for this patient who clearly needed a higher level of care.

As a critical-care paramedic, you have to make a decision on whether your patient is stable enough for transport. In many ways, this patient was not; however, I was provided the resources to safely transport this patient, with the assistance of an ED nurse and a respiratory therapist, and I opted to go on a hellish ride. Sadly, the patient expired, but not due to lack of effort.

7

Placebo Effect

As paramedics, we have committed to an ethical code of "do no harm to your patients." We also have to understand and respect that we are unlicensed professionals who receive orders from medical control either through standing orders or via real-time medical control at a receiving facility.

Do we always abide by the rules? Of course not! We bend them, mend them, and smash them at times. However, I trust myself and my partners to only do so to advance medical care for our patients.

Some time ago, we responded to a reported bee sting with anaphylaxis not too far from our medic station.

Upon arrival at the scene and getting a sense of the situation, we quickly noticed that this male patient was a bit of a hypochondriac and deserved an Oscar for acting out all the symptoms of anaphylaxis without actually having a single one.

To settle his anxieties and demand for an Epi shot, we administered 0.3 mL of normal saline and sent him on his way to the hospital basic life support (BLS).

We thought this was the end of the call until we received that dreaded phone call from our medical control physician demanding that we report to him immediately.

He looked us in the eyes as we were shaking in our boots and simply but forcefully asked, "What in the world did you do?"

After pleading our case, we got away with a slap on our wrists and clear instructions that, although creative, placebos have *no* role in EMS!

8

Where Is Waldo?

Have you ever seen one of those "Where's Waldo?" cartoon drawings? I'm sure you have, and it's often difficult to find that little guy.

You might be scratching your head right about now and wondering how this relates to being a paramedic!

Have you ever been to a busy accident scene in the evening hours under dim lighting with many different disciplines working shoulder to shoulder to rescue an accident victim? Try finding your partner in this crowd. It's difficult unless, of course, you were prepared for this type of a scenario.

For the first three years as flight medics, we wore bright-red jumpsuits, and it was rather easy to pick us out of a crowd or to find your partner in your peripheral vision. For the last two years of my flight career, we wore dark-blue flight suits, allowing us to blend in with fire, police, and EMS personnel.

It truly felt like we'd lost a tool in our fight to provide excellence in care. The moral of this story is the fact that we need to make sure that we wear proper identification, whether it's a badge, ID, patches, or vest plus other unique identifying markers that allow you to stand out in a crowd.

Paramedics should not be camouflaged. Instead, we should be pillars of leadership and easily recognized in the middle of mayhem.

Be seen or be forgotten!

9

They Put That GPS in This Truck for a Reason!

I still smile when I think back before the days of GPS. Someone had painstakingly described every possible response scenario from each of our stations to each road in our primary response area.

It must have taken that person weeks to get this done right. As a user, I can say with great certainty that many lives were affected by this effort, allowing us to shave minutes off our response times. Time is tissue!

Fast-forward to having twenty-first-century equipment in our current emergency response vehicles. With a touch of a few buttons, a friendly voice will tell us where to go step by step. That is, of course, if you bother to use this handy tool.

Time is tissue (lack of oxygen to the brain caused immediate cell death, which worsens survival over time), and regardless of the original dispatch information, minutes can count even in the calls that seem most benign from first description.

Don't get caught with your pants down, something that has happened to me on several occasions. You think you know where you are going and don't bother to use technology to verify, only to find out that you responded to Smith Street when you should have gone to Smit Road.

As we make technological advances in health care, utilize those advances to assist you in getting to the right address or making the right diagnosis.

Right place, right time because time = tissue!

10

EMS Humor

EMS = ExtraMarital Sex or EMS = Easy Money Sleeping! It all sounds like fun to us, but not to everybody. EMS humor has a time and place—just *never* in front of our patients, families, or friends.

We often use humor as a way to debrief and de-stress, which is a perfectly good way to get yourself centered. However, it should not come at the cost of someone else's dignity.

On too many occasions I have certainly been guilty of this, especially in my early years as a paramedic. Let me give you a couple of examples to learn from.

You respond to a cardiac arrest only to find out upon arrival that the patient is an obvious DOA (dead on arrival). No big deal to you, right? A little paperwork and you are on your way again. On such calls, we often end up lingering outside the house with other responders, laughing, joking, and having a good time chatting about whatever.

Sounds perfectly good from our perspective. However, from the perspective of the family members of the deceased, who are in different stages of grieving, it is totally inappropriate and even angering to see responders joking outside their home while they are coming to terms with a tragic loss.

The same can be said of when we are working a scene and we start commenting about the patient—thinking that he or she can't hear us—only to find out the patient heard every word we said.

EMS humor has its place—and for good reason—but we just need to be mindful of where it is done!

11

EMS Love

Love is in the air! We can sense it all around. It's inescapable at all times, and nothing wrong can be said with endless hugs and kisses. It sounds all so romantic and desirable. Right?

EMS love is not an isolated phenomenon. It is something I have seen many times over the past twenty-five years of service. I guess it's what happens when you get like-minded people together with lots of time on their hands in between calls.

Not too long ago, I saw a wedding anniversary announcement on Facebook that my friends were celebrating seventeen years of marriage. It made me smile and laugh out loud, knowing how tumultuous their EMS love affair was.

He was one of my paramedic partners, and she was a great volunteer EMT. On more nights than one, we had to surveil her whereabouts as one didn't trust the other. I'm still flabbergasted about the fact that I participated in this nonsense, but I guess that as a great partner you have to assist your partner in finding great love.

Long story short, it all worked out, and they are now married with two beautiful kids and living a great life, doing what they do best.

Love is everywhere, as it is in EMS too. You will meet some of the most wonderful doctors, nurses, paramedics, and EMTs of the opposite sex, or of the same sex for that matter.

You will find happiness when you are not looking for it, as I did when I met my second wife, Erica, an awesome ED nurse with the softest elbows ever.

12

Volunteers

You can't live with them, and you can't live without them. Knowing that this book will have a wide audience, some of you might have no experience with volunteers while others of you may be embedded within the volunteer services.

No matter if you are a paid paramedic or just volunteering your time, we have to tip our hats to those of you who give up endless hours to provide a service to your community.

Some are great, but many just have a big heart and very few skills. This can be frustrating at times but can also be delightful for the opportunities it presents. You never know who this volunteer is; they can be senior executives, schoolteachers, or local mechanics.

Regardless of who they are or what they do, each has joined a volunteer service to contribute to the community—they never leave home to do intentional harm. Though they can be frustrating beyond belief, they can also be helpful and knowledgeable in such a way that will make a difference in a clinical outcome.

As a *Positude* Paramedic (at least that is how I have positioned myself over the years), it is important to be collaborative: be a teacher, a coach, and a mentor. You will make those around you better over time and will reap the benefits of investing your time to train and develop your volunteers.

If all else fails, mitigate risk by assigning them benign duties, and pray for the best. By far, the majority of my volunteer experiences have been absolutely positive, and I found volunteers to be teachable, respectful, and grateful for your mentorship along the way.

13

Working with the Flight Crew!

As a paramedic, at times you have to call in the troops to assist you with a particularly messy scene, such as a complex extrication from a car or a ravine. Resources might include the fire department, police department, or medivac helicopter.

Frequently, even before you arrive, first responders will make the call to get a medivac to transport a patient to a regional trauma center. However, it is going to be your decision whether to utilize them or not.

Adrenaline rushing, you need to make decisions within minutes of your arrival. You question first responders and assess the situation before making the radio call to confirm the need for medivac transportation.

Not knowing all of the facts, you will at times make the wrong call and send a fractured ankle to the trauma center via medivac. We have all done this and learned from it.

There's a role for medivac transportation, as I experienced while flying for about five years; however, never lose sight of the risk involved. As the lead medic, you reserve the right to cancel the flight crew at any time.

I can tell you with confidence that most flight crews are absolutely fantastic and will gladly assist you in any way possible. Most of them have worked as paramedics for many years and understand the difficulties of being the first to arrive.

Make the right decisions at the right time!

14

Too Nauseated to Fly

It was a dark night from hell. Even writing about it makes me nauseous. Let's give it a try, and I will keep a barf bag nearby just in case.

It all started like a normal shift on the medivac helicopter. I was bantering around with my RN partner and one of the best helicopter pilots I've ever known.

It was a very windy night with gusts up to forty knots and low ceilings at twenty-five hundred feet. We turned in at about 11:00 p.m., hoping for a good night's sleep.

It all ended when we got the call about a car that had rolled off the Tappan Zee Bridge near midspan and was trapped on a pylon. Without hesitation, our pilot accepted the flight to provide light over the accident scene using our very powerful searchlight located on the belly of our aircraft.

It was my turn to be in the back, which isolates you from having any forward vision and leaves you alone in pitch-black darkness. Under normal circumstances this is pleasant and peaceful; however, with forty-knot winds and gusts even greater than that, it is sheer hell.

I remember hovering or bouncing around for about forty-five minutes. It was the longest forty-five minutes ever. I was nauseated from the second I lost any visual reference and felt the aircraft sway from side to side and then bounce up and down and forward and backward.

I could not wait to get my feet back on the ground, and when I finally did a few hours later, I packed my bag and went home, not caring if I ever flew again!

15

Flight Medicine Rules

It is every little boy's dream to fly on a helicopter and rescue the victims of grave accidents. OK, maybe not everybody's dream, but it was mine.

Ever since becoming a paramedic in 1993, I had my eye on that coveted job as a flight paramedic with *STAT* Flight.

It wasn't until they finally changed their flight-crew configuration from two RNs to an RN and a paramedic that my dream job could become a reality.

It seemed like it wasn't meant to be from day one. Some of my experienced partners got hired before I even had a chance to be considered. I never lost the desire; I just had to wait for my turn and be in the right place at the right time.

I finally got my chance to join the team in 2003 and flew for five years, primarily out of Westchester Medical Center or a remote base in Kobelt, New York.

Flying and medicine is a perfect combination, and it will challenge you both mentally and physically. It was worth every minute of my time, even though the compensation was not commensurate with the risk associated with flying in a helicopter.

The many hours of rounding, observing, participating, and learning from the brightest doctors, nurses, and respiratory therapists in the PICU, ICCU, ICU, TICU, and NICU were exceptional.

I miss flying every day and compensate for it by continuing to work as a 911 medic and flying my own fixed-wing Piper Warrior II whenever I get a chance.

Never give up on your dream!

16

Going Above and Beyond

The title of this chapter might make you think of the heroic efforts that are made at trauma scenes. However, in this case, it is more about what we as *Positude* Paramedics do every day by going above and beyond for our patients.

Peter was one of our long-time frequent flyers in our system. He was a fragile diabetic and, whenever he was hypoglycemic, a royal pain in the ass.

When awake, conscious, and alert, Peter was one of the most caring and friendly individuals you will ever meet.

Not because he was special but rather because he absolutely refused to go to the hospital for his hypoglycemic episodes, we frequently treated and released him after his blood sugar was within normal limits.

Well, that's what our goal is for most of our diabetic patients, but Peter was a bit different. He demanded more from us.

We made an agreement with Peter to never transport him unless it was absolutely warranted, and we agreed to not only bring his blood sugar back within normal limits but that we would prepare his food to prevent a secondary hypoglycemia, which can be devastating to the patient.

There were weeks we went to his house two to three times per week, fought with him to get glucagon on board, and then dined with him afterward to ensure he got some complex carbs into him.

This is going above and beyond on a normal day in the life of a *Positude* Paramedic. I miss Peter!

17

The Honor to Save a Life

There are a few things in life you will never forget besides the birth of your own children.

After losing the battle to save a child from cardiac arrest, you will wonder forever about what else you could have done.

On the opposite side of the spectrum, you will never forget the lives you saved where patients returned to normal activities and got to enjoy their families once again.

It is truly an honor that is bestowed upon us as well as a tremendous responsibility to have the abilities to save a life.

To save a life, a chain of events must be executed flawlessly to improve the chances of a positive outcome.

Over the span of my career, I have been fortunate to be part of such chains of events that led to outcomes that extended the lives of both the very young and the old.

I got to witness them when their EKG flatlined, their eyes sunken, and their soul about to depart. I got to be part of their graduations, weddings, and family celebrations. In actuality, my youngest save ever, whom I consider my little brother, is making the most out of his life and is now giving back as a registered nurse.

It truly is an honor to save a life. Not too many people can ever say they've done that. Be proud of your abilities and stay sharp because you never know when it is your turn to have the honor to save a life.

18

Friends for Life

Some people ask me what is the difference between an office job and being a paramedic. Where to start? There are so many differences, but none more significant than the fact that you are glued to a partner twelve to twenty-four hours at a time.

I suppose it could also be the longest day ever if you don't like your partner or work with someone who smells, smokes, farts, or snores so loud that the station rattles.

However, when things click and there's chemistry, it is a great opportunity to build friendships for life.

I grew up in Holland with two sisters, but I longed for a big brother.

Over the past twenty-five years in EMS, I have not only gained a bigger brother but have adopted several little brothers and sisters as well.

I'm so incredibly lucky to work with some of the very best paramedics whom I call my friends. We are friends for life, even if we don't speak every day or take family trips together.

Our bond is our passion for our patients, quality care and safety of patients and sharing our craft with the next generation.

I promise you that I rarely hear this from my friends in the finance or business world.

Take care of your partners, and they will take care of you!

19

My Work Wife

It all started about eighteen years ago at Rockland Paramedic Service Medic 3 Station where I was a station lieutenant at that time. I met my work wife Bernadette, and life has not been the same since.

Bern is actually seven days older than I am, but she will tell you that she is years wiser and at least a decade younger looking.

Right from day one, we formed a strong and lasting bond. We were able to work together on complex medical or trauma cases without wondering what the other was going to do next. Although important, it is not the reason why we bonded.

We worked together, got to know each other on a deep personal level, and cared for each other through the happiness of childbirth and the sadness of my divorce. We enjoyed endless talks about the future and tried every possible diet until we finally gave up and learned to accept me for me.

I'm genuinely a better person because of Bern—she will tell me how it is without hesitation but with a caring heart. I know in my heart that many of our patients have benefited from our common bond and common understanding.

If you have the opportunity to work with an awesome partner for years to come, I highly recommend it. I truly got lucky in more ways than one.

20

Fourteen Jobs in Twelve Hours

It's 6:00 p.m. I have been working for the past eleven hours and finally see the light at the end of the tunnel.

It's been a hard day right out of the gate. Nonstop since early morning, we treated depression, lacerations, chest pain, a couple fall victims, an emotionally disturbed person (EDP), and a choking victim.

It's only 6:00 p.m., with another hour to go, and I still have to write and log eleven prehospital care reports.

Hoping my relief will come in early (but that rarely happens anymore), I heard the tones sound and our dispatcher give the instructions for the next job.

I felt like kicking something but I was too tired to do so. Nearly worn out, we got back in the truck and responded to a Code 3. We were not even halfway there before our dispatcher requested us to split for job number thirteen.

I dropped off my partner and responded to fall victim number three for the day. Luckily, a BLS unit arrived just before I did and canceled me before making patient contact.

Breathing a big sigh of relief, I made a right turn toward base. It was 6:35 p.m. I could smell the end of my shift, but it wasn't long before the tones went off again and that horrible voice on the other end dispatched us to a cardiac arrest due to a heroin overdose.

I was shot, my night was shot, and I had little energy left. Did I mention it was nearly one hundred degrees outside with dense humidity?

I got home drenched, tired, and worn out after fourteen jobs in twelve hours.

21

Sixty-Minute Response Time

How long is too long to respond to a 911 call after you receive your initial dispatch? Great question, and you will find answers that could span from "one minute" to "depending on the type of emergency."

I'm an old-timer and still feel a great sense of pride and urgency as soon as the tones go off, regardless of the type of emergency we were dispatched to.

I do admit that I often need to make a pit stop in the middle of the night before heading out, especially now that I'm getting a little older.

Still, more often than not, I'm in the driver's seat within minutes of dispatch, all too often waiting for minutes before my partners wander in.

There's a direct correlation between the age of the paramedic and the delayed response times. I'm not sure why this is, but I don't remember being like this when I had just started.

As a *Positude* Paramedic, take great pride in the fact that you can be ready to respond on a moment's notice. I think that fewer than two minutes during daytime hours and two to three minutes at night is an appropriate standard to maintain.

22

Being Treated by Your Best Friend

A few years ago, I sat in my favorite chair in our medic station where I had fallen asleep many times before. At the crack of dawn, I awoke a bit confused, wondering why I never went to bed.

After regaining my senses, I stretched my extremities to loosen up the joints before I could get up. I'm not sure what happened, but I felt something that was not quite normal.

I suddenly had this sunken feeling, a bit of heaviness in my chest, and soon thereafter I broke out in a cold sweat. After connecting the dots, I realized that I caused a Valsalva from stretching while sitting in my chair.

It only took a few minutes for my heart rate to come up, but this time it didn't stay within normal limits. Instead, it got faster and faster until it got stuck on about two hundred beats per minute.

Initially, I was in denial but soon realized that I needed to wake up my partner and best friend to seek treatment for this sudden SVT (supraventricular tachycardia). As she will tell you, I was the worst patient ever.

Before getting onto the stretcher, I insisted on going to the bathroom and wanted to call medical control myself. Although I wasn't short of breath or had any chest pain, I needed to go to the hospital to convert my supraventricular tachycardia back to a normal sinus rhythm.

My partner did everything right while as a patient I did everything wrong. Thank you, Bern, for treating me that night, and I apologize for having been a pain in the A!

23

Growing Up Together

I'm twenty years older but I never grew up, just got grayer, heavier, and crankier at 2:00 a.m., when the tones go off one more time. Mentally, I'm still twenty-five years old, although that's not completely true anymore either.

I was a young man when I started in EMS. I thought that forty-five-year-olds were over the hill for this young person's job.

You know what is exciting and amazing about the world of emergency services? We start young and grow older together. By nature, we are loyal not only to our profession but to our partners.

We are creatures of habit, and once you find the right work partner, we tend to latch on and go for the ride.

I have been around the same group of guys and gals for over twenty years. We have laughed, cried, and cheered together. We have been through death, divorces, marriages, and childbirth together.

Most importantly, we got wiser together as our bodies got older and our souls matured. We have had the opportunity to be there for one another, to watch our kids play together, and to mentor the next generation.

There's camaraderie and sometimes even love—growing up together with my friends doing the job we love most is truly a privilege.

24

A Patient Complaint

During twenty-five years of responding to medical emergencies all across New York State, I must have had twenty thousand or more patient contacts in that period of time. I can't recall 90 percent of the calls; however, I can remember 100 percent of the complaints I have ever received.

Even though I have only received two official patient complaints against me, I remember each scenario like it was yesterday.

The first one happened nearly two decades ago, at which time I was accused of not treating a trauma patient correctly by failing to do an EKG.

The second complaint was not too long ago. I was accused of being rude, impatient, and not empathetic toward my patient.

It still hurts to think that someone felt so strongly about my care that they followed through by filing a complaint.

What was I to do? I could go straight into denial mode, or I could be reflective and introspective about the complaint that was brought to my attention.

Over my careers as a student, teacher, mentor, and coach, I have always taken a step back to reflect on the situation and to put myself in the shoes of the patient.

Although I was not clinically wrong in my decision, taking an EKG would not have harmed this patient and maybe would have settled the nerves of the daughter.

I was dead wrong in the second complaint. I have learned from that situation and will never make that mistake again.

25

On Your Own

Let's go back to 1992 in rural Hancock, New York, which is about 140 miles northwest of New York City in the middle of nowhere. At least it felt like that more often than not.

Boomer and I had just graduated from our EMT critical-care course and were the first to provide advanced life-support services at this level in our rural little town.

The nearest trauma center was located in Binghamton, New York, only fifty minutes away while going Code 3.

We had no cell phones and no UHF or VHF communications with medical control—just basic guidelines and a prayer to get us there in one piece.

One day we got a request for a young man in respiratory distress. Upon arrival, we found him in status asthmaticus, shutting down in front of our eyes.

What was even worse, it was one of Boomer's childhood friends, and we had worked on his father as a cardiac-arrest case only weeks before.

We did all we could to save his life but to no avail. We felt like we were all on our own, that there was nobody else to consult on what else we could do. We drove as fast as we could, but things didn't look good. It took nearly an hour to get to Binghamton General Hospital only to hear the emergency-room doctor pronounce him dead upon arrival.

I was grateful that I was there with and for my friend Boomer and feel in my heart that we did all we could have done. It's one of those calls that will stick with me forever.

26

Great Partners

What makes a great partner? Is it someone who talks a lot or speaks very little, or is it one who snores or watches TV all night? The answer is pretty simple: not unlike a good marriage, it all depends on you as an individual.

What is it that you need in a partner, and what is it that you are willing to do for your partner?

Go back to one of the key drivers to long-term success: Work hard to build synergistic relationships with your partners. Get to know them, pay attention to their intrinsic drivers, and be genuine in your caring.

Personally, I look for partners whom I can converse with, someone who appreciates a good conversation, who is honest, direct in feedback about life, relationships, and clinical care.

I'm an alpha dog who has learned to follow other alpha dogs to prevent any discord. If and when possible, I'm the first to the truck, first into the scene, and the first to start aggressive treatment.

I have been very lucky in my partner selections over the years. It always worked even though it took some time to gel with a few of them.

I value a great partner, and so should you. Together you can accomplish more and improve clinical outcomes.

To find a great partner, you need to be an awesome partner.

27

What Is This Medication?

If you make it a goal to memorize fifty medications per day for the next one hundred days, you will be the perfect paramedic...said nobody ever.

Physicians, who are the primary prescribers of medications, only really know the top one hundred medications that they frequently prescribe. After many years of practicing and studying, they will possess a mental database of about five hundred medications but will still rely on their *Physician's Desk Reference* to find the right dosing and frequency.

As a *Positude* Paramedic, I have a working knowledge of about fifty medications and will still have to reference an app to identify a medication's actions, interactions, and side effects. Nothing to be ashamed about. It's impossible to know it all.

What is possible is that if you are not completely honest with yourself, you'll become complacent, arrogant, and unsafe in your practice of providing care to your patients.

Whenever you go to a scene with a patient with a slew of chronic diseases, you should expect a boatload of medications including but not limited to prescriptions, vitamins, herbal supplements, and foreign pills that contain who knows what.

Adopt a golden rule for yourself: *never* allow a patient to take his or her medications unless you are familiar with the drug.

As a *Positude* Paramedic, you will become a master of resource management and will adapt your means to whatever the situation calls for. Know that you are never alone, and there are lots of smart people standing by to assist in making the right decisions for your patients.

28

Calling Poison Control

Where is your umbrella when you need it? Always in the opposite place of where it needs to be. The same can be said for important resources or telephone numbers: they are rarely thought of when they should be utilized.

The most likely scenario where you would utilize poison control is a pediatric emergency call where a patient swallowed an unknown substance or pills. You might be familiar with the medication; however, it is unlikely that you will know how it acts on a pediatric patient or if it was potentiated by other medications.

One of the most dangerous overdoses you have to be mindful about is a Tylenol OD in pediatric patients. It can have a deadly effect and/or cause damage for life.

Google "Poison Control" plus your region and store the number in your cell phone. Now you will be ready without delay.

As a *Positude* Paramedic, make sure you keep this number both in your cell phone and written on a Post-it that you keep securely in your wallet. Do it right now!

You should also make it a point to photograph any chemicals, capsules, or pills found at the scene. If possible and safe, bring samples of what was taken accidentally or on purpose to the hospital for further investigation.

Don't overlook accidental overdoses by our geriatric patient population. Take your time to look over their medication regimen, and calculate the number of pills left against the medication's prescription date.

Poison lurks everywhere, so remain suspicious at all times.

29

Another Motorcycle Accident

The sun is cresting over the horizon, birds are singing, and blossoms are blooming. It's that time of the year again, spring—also known as motorcycle accident season.

It is as predictable as the sun rising in the morning!

As a 911 paramedic, I saw my fair share of motorcycle accidents, but it paled in comparison to my years flying on a medivac helicopter.

It seemed an almost daily occurrence that we would respond to a motorcycle accident with significant injuries. Often it was too late, and other times we picked up bodies rather than people with significant injuries.

Their bodies were devastated by traumatic injuries such as flail chest, eviscerations, open-book fractures, and many distracting extremity fractures.

Not knowing what you will find, be prepared for the absolute worst and don't blindly trust what the patient relates back to you. Use a high index of suspicion when examining the scene, the helmet, and the motorcycle itself.

Treat for the worst-case scenario and pray for the best. Be mindful that you don't get caught up with treating distracting injuries like a mangled extremity while the patient bleeds to death.

Personally, I could live without ever seeing another motorcycle victim, especially those who just want to ride for pure joy and get wiped out by a driver who is not paying attention.

30

On My Way to a DOA!

I can tell you that over the past twenty-plus years, I have completely changed my viewpoint about my response to a cardiac arrest or DOA.

In my younger years, I saw cardiac-arrest patients as opportunities to practice my skills, with the hope of saving a life.

Over many years, I started looking at this from a different angle and suddenly saw a loving father, mother, sister, or brother who didn't need to be poked, probed, or assaulted with machines, tubes, and IVs.

That doesn't mean I won't work a code—I just use all my clinical skills, judgment, and consultation with my partners or medical control to determine how to best proceed.

When appropriate, we stop resuscitation and transition to caring for and comforting the family. It was not until I buried my father—who was viewed at home and never went to the morgue—that I appreciated the importance of spending time with your loved one in your home environment rather than being in a busy, loud, disruptive emergency room to say your last good-byes.

Today, I will take the time to clean up the scene, place the deceased back into bed, prop up their heads, cover their bodies, and present them to their families.

I have yet to receive a single complaint and truly hope that these last experiences bring comfort and hope to those left behind to grieve.

31

Last Message to My Family
on September 11, 2001

I remember that day like it was yesterday. I can retrace every step from receiving the initial news, the all-call back to HQ, and the manic drive down Route 17 at unsafe speeds.

While driving down, I saw lots of FDNY firefighters and NYPD officers making the same trip down toward New York City. I remember coming around the corner on the New York State Thruway in Suffern, New York—it was a crystal-clear day, allowing you to see Lower Manhattan from about thirty miles away.

I could clearly see at least one tower ablaze. At that time on that dreadful day in September 2001, none of us would have thought that both towers would be gone by midday.

After arriving at HQ, we gathered and waited for our assignments, not knowing what was going to happen next.

This was not the time to respond into NYC and freelance. It was time to organize, prepare, and ready ourselves to respond to wherever they needed us to go.

Over the next few hours, it became crystal clear to all of us that we were at war, with multiple sites being hit at the same time. This restricted our movements to ensure we had the west side of the Hudson River covered just in case.

Finally we got the call to mobilize, which left each of us to make that last call home. I remember my voice quavering, not knowing what the day would bring. I made it home that day; however, too many did not.

Make your last words count—you just never know.

32

How Many Jobs Do I Need to Support My Family?

My eight-year-old son Max will ask me from time to time if I'm rich. The answer is simply "Yes, filthy rich. Not monetarily but in love!" Max often replies by saying that he is rich too.

I started working as a paramedic in 1993 at eleven dollars per hour—nothing great, but in comparison to medics in the northern part of New York State who were earning only seven dollars an hour, I thought I had riches and was grateful for the opportunity.

I wish I had a choice, but I really didn't have one back then. If I wanted to put enough food on the table and pay my rent, I needed to work at least sixty to eighty hours per week.

Sadly, even though wages have gone up over the past twenty-three years, a paramedic's starting pay is still not enough to support a family of four. We have lots of work to do to bring pay parity among paramedics to a level where it can support a family, but it won't come without a struggle.

Today, being a paramedic is still more about being mission driven and wanting to make a difference in someone's life than it is about being a real career.

However, there's hope for the future, and lots of good folks are working on a better future for paramedics. I have never regretted becoming a paramedic, even with all the pain, hardship, and time away from my family.

33

Lifelong Commitment

Receiving specialized medical training is truly a commitment for life. Forever going forward, you will feel the duty to step up to the plate whenever someone calls for help. You know Murphy's Law: the call for duty will always come when you're least prepared or when it's the most inconvenient.

I remember once I was flying back from San Francisco to Washington, DC. As I boarded the plane, I noticed an elderly lady in the front of the aircraft who wasn't looking so hot, and I had a fleeting thought about her medical condition en route.

Some four hours into the flight, when we were crossing the state line from Ohio into Pennsylvania, the call for assistance was made on the overhead speaker, asking if there was a doctor on board.

My earlier fleeting thoughts became a reality as I found the same elderly lady unresponsive, cool, and clammy on the floor in front of her seat.

Utilizing the equipment available, I applied oxygen, placed her in a supine position with elevated legs, and inserted an IV for fluid administration. As she slowly regained consciousness, the pilot asked me if I wanted to divert to Pittsburgh, Pennsylvania, to get our patient to the nearest hospital or continue for another forty minutes and land at our final destination.

All I wanted was to catch my connecting flight, and I felt my patient was stable enough to make it home herself. Upon arrival, our patient was whisked off to the hospital and I walked away with a nice bottle of wine and an upgrade on the next flight. When duty calls, a *Positude* Paramedic responds.

34

Mouth-to-Mouth Resuscitation

The last time anybody should have done mouth-to-mouth resuscitation without a mask would have been in the early '80s, before the AIDS epidemic started.

Sadly, many didn't pay attention and continued the old practices of poor utilization of personal protective equipment (PPE). Although not immediately evident, many have gotten sick with hepatitis A, B, and C or HIV/AIDS. Most were exposed to these diseases by trying to save a life and by their own negligence to protect themselves first and rescue others second.

I'm the first to admit that I have not been the best at wearing PPE, especially not my latex gloves. I depend on the feeling in my fingertips to sense the skin, feel a pulse, or palpate a vein when starting an IV.

Every time I violate this rule, I expose myself to the unknown, and I expose my wife, kids, and others to the potential of a deadly germ.

Just like doing mouth-to-mouth resuscitation without a medium is a thing of the past, touching patients without wearing gloves should also not be an option.

Handwashing with water and soap or just using hand sanitizer is the minimum you can do for yourself and your family.

An ounce of prevention is worth its weight in gold!

35

Lucas CPR Device

After twenty-five-plus years in the business, I always wondered about ways to provide effective CPR without breaking our backs. I considered many things but never anything good enough for production.

After I thought I had seen it all, the good old thumper made a comeback after a complete overhaul. Meet Lucas, the most effective chest compression machine ever made.

You want to know how effective this thing is? Let me tell you a short but shocking story.

I once found an elderly gentleman at the bottom of his stairs in cardiac arrest. According to his wife, it had happened only ten minutes ago. Luckily we were ready to go with our Lucas device and applied it within minutes of arrival.

After I intubated the patient, now ten minutes later, we transferred him to our awaiting ambulance. With a couple rounds of Epinephrine on board, our patient suddenly opened his eyes and tried to communicate with us. I immediately stopped the Lucas device to check for a pulse.

Much to my chagrin, as soon as I turned off the device, so did the patient. Initially, it didn't make any sense since I had never seen this before. The Lucas device was so effective that it had essentially replaced his nonfunctional heart.

Needless to say, I didn't turn off the device again, and even in the hospital they had a hard time deciding to continue or to count on the Lucas device to give the patient any hope. In the end, it was false hope as his heart was totally shot, but it gave the patient's wife the opportunity to say good-bye.

36

MAST Trouser

I have always promised myself that the day that sodium bicarbonate becomes a first-line cardiac-arrest drug that I would quit on the spot. It is absolutely amazing to see the changes in clinical care over time.

MAST trousers, although a great idea, never panned out in EMS as it was originally thought they would.

Only second to spider straps, MAST trousers are the single most confusing tool to apply in a crisis situation.

Over the years, we have applied them for two clinical indications and have only really noticed a benefit in one of those cases.

The typical indication for using MAST trousers was hypovolemic shock. It took foresight, practice, and lots of extra hands to apply them, inflate them, and monitor for uncontrolled external bleeding not suppressed by the trousers. Although not scientific, it rarely improved the clinical or dynamic measures.

However, I still believe that MAST trousers could or should play a role in long-bone femur fractures and open-book pelvic fractures. I used them in both types of scenarios and found they stabilized the fractures, improved comfort, and reduced pain for our patients.

Just like a venturi mask, MAST trousers have fallen out of favor due to their complexity and their unproven clinical benefits versus the other options available.

I guess we could donate our MAST trousers to the Air National Guard to use when flying high-performance aircraft.

37

I Got Hit by a Billy Club!

In many ways, we have been lucky and a bit spoiled in our three-tiered response system. Every time someone calls 911 in our township, two police officers, two medics, and an ambulance respond to the scene. It's a luxury, and it does provide a sense of security and an extra resource just in case.

Working with our colleagues who carry guns and billy clubs brings another dimension to relationship building, especially when working nights with the same guys for the past twenty-plus years.

One in particular stands out: an aspiring actor himself, Dan is a bear of a guy and at fifty is still one of the strongest guys on the force. Just ask him and he will tell you.

Part of our stress-relief efforts is bantering with the cops and exchanging friendly insults.

One particularly dark night, we were the first to arrive at the scene. As we were trying to size up the scene, I didn't pay much attention to what was coming from behind.

All in good fun, Dave had snuck up and suddenly nailed me on the back of my knees with his billy club, causing them to buckle and nearly causing me to eat dirt.

What does Mom always tell you? "It's all good and well until someone gets hurt!"

In actuality, although painful initially, we have shared a special bond ever since.

Without a single doubt, I know he will have our back at any time, and that's what really matters after all.

38

My Fifteen-Pound Cell Phone

Recently, we were driving around in Adirondack Park in Upstate New York and saw an old-fashioned phone booth. I asked my kids if they knew what this booth was for. After some hesitation, my son, Max, told me that it was a place to go pee! Not far from the truth, right?

It is absolutely amazing to see the technological advances that have come about in our lifetime. We have seen computers shrink from a size of a room to something so small that you hold it with just one hand. We now know that an iPad has enough computer power to do the job of all the computers in the original space shuttle.

In EMS, we have gone from a bulky thirty-pound suitcase with a UHF radio to a fifteen-pound bag containing a telephone to now a barely four-ounce smartphone that can be activated through a watch. What is next? These are exciting times.

Telemedicine is next. Similar to body cameras for our police officers, paramedics will soon have the ability to telecommunicate with medical control through secure videoconferencing.

This is, of course, less important in densely populated areas with several hospitals nearby. However, it could be a lifesaver if you have a sixty-minute or longer ride to the hospital.

Telemedicine is intended not to take away paramedics' current decision-making process but to enhance their abilities to treat and release. I mentioned this in my opening chapters and feel strongly that the future of paramedicine is going to be distinctively different, just like how we have advanced from our fifteen-pound cell-phone bag.

39

Rural Paramedicine

If you think it is tough to climb an eight-story walk-up apartment building in a big city, think about your colleagues who have response times in excess of hours and embark into wilderness areas to retrieve their patients.

In reality, both are tough and exciting at the same time. Each comes with unique concerns for safety and physical demands.

Part of being a *Positude* Paramedic is to be ready for the unknown, to be on top of your game, and to be nimble in your response regardless of location and access to resources such as medical control or the Internet.

Personally, when I worked in Delaware County, New York, we had regular response times of over twenty minutes, and it took sixty-plus minutes to get to a local hospital.

We relied upon forest rangers and medivac helicopters to decrease the time in getting from the place of the incident to the emergency room. What is considered a moderate injury in an urban location, such as a dislocated hip or fractured femur, is a critical injury in a rural location. Time equals tissue—minor bleeding over a sixty-minute period adds up to significant volume loss.

Being a rural paramedic is exciting in its own right: you are likely the sole medical professional, and both your team and your patients rely on your professionalism and abilities to get them to definitive treatment.

40

Intubation versus CPAP

There was a time before CPAP when every patient in acute pulmonary edema and every COPD patient struggling for air needed to be intubated to receive ventilator support.

There are two significant changes in the science of medicine that have changed the way we practice today and the types of patients we see.

I'm basing the following on profound personal experiences and not scientific proof.

The improvements in effective steroidal inhalers have significantly decreased medical emergencies among asthmatics and COPD patients. We used to respond to such calls on a daily basis, but today I can't remember the last asthma or COPD patient I saw.

Although management of CHF (congestive heart failure) with combination medication and left ventricular–assist devices has decreased the incidence of acute episodes, we still see a fair share of these patients.

In the past, we needed to intubate these patients in order to save their lives, causing significant issues with weaning them off the ventilators in the days and weeks thereafter. This comes at a very high cost to both the patient and the hospital.

Finally, after years of clinical trials, CPAP was introduced to EMS and life changed for both the paramedics and the patients alike.

We apply CPAP and miracles happen!

41

How Many Pints of Blood Do We Have?

"Not enough" is the real answer! Just ask any patient with an arterial bleed, a leaking aneurism, or major trauma.

We have yet to find the perfect solution to prehospital hemorrhaging in regard to replacement. We have seen improvements in tourniquets, Quickclot gauze, and other devices that assist with external bleeding. Direct pressure, elevation, and rapid transport make up the BLS version of bleeding prevention bleeding, and it still works well in many scenarios.

I will never forget a 911 call on State Route 17 in Monticello, New York. A brilliant young volleyball player returning from a tournament lost control of her vehicle and wrapped it around the center column of an overhead sign. Although technically alive, she was unresponsive and bleeding profusely only from her head.

We quickly stabilized her but had no way to control her bleeding, so we opted to take her to the local hospital instead of the nearest trauma center some forty minutes away.

She needed blood products and lots of them to have a fighting chance of recovery. We made a quick turnaround from the local hospital and were en route with a rapid transfusion of blood. I believe that we used three to four pints plus lots of Lactate Ringers as well. With blood dripping from the back steps, her hemorrhaging was out of control.

It's most likely that she clinically died at the scene, but we worked hard to preserve her organs. Her parents graciously donated them for others to have the gift of life.

42

The Gift of Life

I hope that you read the previous story before starting this one. I'm still saddened by what happened that day and have seen this play out many times since, but not always with the preferred ending of giving someone the "gift of life."

Setting aside any religious or cultural justification for not donating one's organs to either science or life, we need to do more to make a difference.

I'm not going to cite the statistics since they can easily be found through a Google search. I'm going to focus on the need to be aware as *Positude* Paramedics of when we treat our patients and/or when we discuss end of life with family and friends.

Thinking about organ donation for the first time when an incident occurs is not particularly helpful. Family members are frequently offended by the thought alone. They are either hopeful for a miracle or in denial.

We (health-care professionals) need to make end-of-life, health-care proxy, MOLST, and DNR/DNI organ donation part of our active discussion. We should lead by example by signing the reverse of our driver's licenses to indicate that we are willing to donate our organs just in case.

I have had the good fortune of being part of several occasions when donor families were introduced to the recipient families. It is the purest joy I have ever seen.

To hear the heartbeat of your late son, father, or brother or your daughter, mother, or sister providing vital life to the recipient is powerful. It's instantly gratifying to know that he or she gets to live on and provide life.

43

My First Baby

There are a few things in the life of a paramedic that you want to do but preferably should never have to do. Childbirth in a nonhospital setting is one of those things.

There's nothing more gratifying if it all goes as designed; however, if things don't go well, it can be, and often is, a disaster you won't ever forget.

Preparation is going to be the key to your success in scenarios such as these. Knowing and understanding the physiology of birth and your equipment will be vital factors in a positive outcome.

I will remember my first delivery forever. The patient was perfect, G4P3 without previous complications; our BLS crew was top notch and well prepared; the environmental temperatures were favorable; and we were ready just in case.

Like most patients under similar circumstances, they will call EMS after their "water breaks" or when their contractions are coming around three to four minutes apart.

Your mind-set should always be to avoid childbirth outside a hospital; however, just like in this case, when the baby wants out, it comes out. Often moms know best, so carefully listen to the words they use.

We were ready, all set up in the back of the ambulance with the hope she could endure the ten-minute ride to the hospital. After hitting the first bump in the road and hearing a yelp from our patient, we knew that the baby was coming and there was no stopping her.

We delivered a beautiful, strong, and healthy baby girl together as a team—a moment in life that we will never forget!

44

Keeping an Eye on You!

I have spent a significant amount of time describing the importance of developing robust partnerships with your paramedic partners, EMTs, police, and firefighters. Partnership actually means being responsible together, having each other's back, offsetting each other's weaknesses, and enduring together, never alone.

This all sounds awesome, especially if you work with someone you trust. However, not everybody can be trusted.

I'm a bit naïve myself from time to time, which prevents me from seeing what I need to see. If you're the same way, know this about yourself and learn to be a bit skeptical. If you don't know how, ask a police officer—this is his or her expertise.

I once had a partner who always knew where the destination address was without verifying or using GPS. On more than one occasion, we arrived late where minutes could have made a difference.

I once had a partner who frequently used narcotics on his patients without making any difference in how the patients perceived their pain level. Although initially he was in denial, we found out that he was giving a fraction of the doses to his patients and keeping the rest for himself.

Keep an eye on your brethren, especially if you work with them infrequently. Liability is shared regardless of who pulled the trigger.

If you see something, say something. It is your responsibility to your patients to ensure safe and quality care.

45

Drug Calculations

Repeat after me: "I'm a mathematic idiot, my life is unmanageable in regard to drug calculation, and I'm rendered powerless. I get hives, an itchy throat, and even hyperventilate when I need to calculate the right medication dose for my patients."

How many of you can relate to this? Most of you will to some extent, though some of you have adopted strategies to help you overcome, and a few of you are mathematical whiz kids and have no clue what I'm making a big deal about.

A few years ago, I responded to a call for a patient with shortness of breath, dizziness, and crushing chest pain. Sounds familiar, right?

Once I found a patient in cardiogenic shock who also had acute pulmonary edema *and* an allergic reaction to an antibiotic that had been borrowed from the patient's wife. What do you do next? What comes first, second, or third?

Thank God that our alphabet starts with ABC or airway, breathing, and circulation. Following this basic logic, our patient was intubated and had an IV started, and now we considered which medication to give first. Epinephrine to counter the anaphylaxis, dopamine versus dobutamine, or load and go to let the ED figure it out?

The smart approach is a quick consultation with medical control to discuss the sequence and dosing of the medications. We decided on Epi 1:1,000 0.3 mL SQ followed by dobutamine drip at 30 gtts/minute. Using our handy chart, we quickly prepared our medications and saw the improvements right in front of our eyes. Resource management saved the day once again.

46

Difficult Intubation

Did you know that the average paramedic today only intubates 1.5 times per year? (Does that mean they only half intubate the second patient?) That is really not enough practice to maintain your competence in this critical skill set.

Over the years, we have seen some technological advances in intubation as equipment has been moving away from the EOA toward the King Air device. The original endotracheal tube has not changed, but advances in blades, lighting, LED, or video equipment have improved our abilities to secure difficult airways.

With any skill you practice, you need to be hyperaware of your personal abilities and your equipment and must always stay two steps ahead of your patient's needs. Redundancy and rescue equipment should be readily available, especially if you opt to use paralytic agents to facilitate intubation.

I have seen some disastrous outcomes both in the field and in a hospital setting due to sheer ignorance and arrogance. I'm hesitant to describe actual scenarios without potentially implicating someone or creating liability for myself.

As a *Positude* Paramedic, you will always strive for safe, quality care, and you will always be prepared with functional equipment and the knowledge of when to use certain devices or medication and, more importantly, when not to use them.

Always remember that the name of this game is oxygen to the brain!

47

Airway Management: A Team Sport

Securing an airway is not a time for heroics—it's the time for competent teamwork to optimize clinical outcomes, safety, and quality in care.

I remember such a scenario from a few years ago. It was a time before every car had airbags, a time when drivers on occasion literally tried eating the steering wheel, causing severe LaForte fractures to their faces that compromised their airways and ability to oxygenate.

One particular patient had a LaForte IV fracture, one of the worst of its kind. His mandible was literally split in half with a compound fracture, causing his tongue to hang onto his neck. His upper dentures were all smashed, with many teeth missing, and his nose and cheekbones were crushed. I identified his airway and looked for bubbles in the back of his throat. How he was still alive was beyond any of us.

It literally took a village to extricate him from his vehicle and place him on the gurney. Up to this point, all we could do was to provide high oxygen by mask, which somehow sustained him until we laid him onto a wooden backboard.

Each person, from the driver, EMT, police officer, firefighter to the paramedic, had a role to play to save his life. Now that he was in the back of the ambulance, it was our turn to play offense. Being prepared and knowledgeable on how to use a boogie, I skipped all the traditional techniques, knowing that his facial structure or lack thereof could not support it. While someone suctioned to keep his airway clear and another stabilized his head to protect the c-spine, I intubated using a boogie, successfully allowing this patient to live another day. Only a *team* could have done this.

48

You Just Didn't, Right?

I was not personally involved in this incident, but it was described to me in great detail. Although the outcome was not preventable, the circumstances in their attempts to save a life still make me smile today.

A 911 call activated the EMS system to respond to a local MRI facility for a patient experiencing an anaphylactic reaction to dye.

Upon arrival, they found an unresponsive middle-aged man in severe respiratory distress with clear signs of facial edema, pulmonary edema, hives, and tachycardia.

Upon initial assessment, it came to be known that the patient's airway was severely compromised and essentially occluded, preventing effective ventilation. Without any significant change after administering Epi SQ, the medics made the decision to perform a needle cricothyrotome.

As the two senior medics worked feverishly to save a life, the entire team of responders worked together to get the equipment set up and to plan for a quick exit.

As one was setting up for the procedure and mentally preparing himself to do something we rarely have to resort to, the other got the right needle of choice and performed the procedure behind his back, much to the surprise of his partner.

They did the very best under very difficult circumstances to save a life that day. What they will remember most is the moment of truth: "You just didn't do that, right?"

49

Making a Mistake

It goes without saying that I have never made a single mistake of any kind. I have never violated a policy, a guideline, or a protocol in my entire career. Right? Wrong, I have done all the above not once but several times.

What will define you as a paramedic over your career is your ability to recognize a mistake and turn it into an opportunity to learn, improve, and strengthen your skills, knowledge, and abilities.

I will describe one such mistake that I learned from. Over the past decade, protocols have changed for the way we treat and where we should transport our trauma, cardiac, and stroke patients.

In this scenario, I was caring for a shortness-of-breath patient with a significant history of COPD who had denied any chest pain at initial contact. After listening to his lung sounds, I developed a care plan based on a working diagnosis of exacerbated COPD and decided to provide conventional treatment as I had done many times before.

I didn't think cardiac; therefore, I didn't do a 12-lead EKG, which would have shown a posterior wall myocardial infarction that I hadn't picked up in the precordial leads. Needless to say, within fifteen minutes of arrival at the local hospital, the acute STEMI protocol was activated, requiring the patient to be transferred to the local STEMI center for definitive treatment.

I could have made many excuses for why I didn't take the EKG. Instead I took responsibility, learned from this event, and made it my goal to perform better in the future.

Failures create opportunities!

50

Cell-Phone Use by Our Patients

Cell phones have become a double-edged sword for sure. They can store vital information including a medication list, diagnosis, treatment, and even EKGs. On the flip side they can be used against us by secretly recording audio or videotaping our conversations and treatment modalities.

It is the new normal, and paramedics have to make the necessary adjustments to safeguard against HIPAA violations.

One of the new norms actually irritates me to no end, but I have little to no influence over changing these behaviors.

I'm sure you can relate to this as well. Whenever you respond to a car accident, most likely all the victims are yapping on their cell phones, preparing their legal cases against the accused.

Only after a firm request will they take the phone from their ears and allow us to ask some basic questions regarding injuries or the mechanism of the incident itself.

At times, I feel like walking away, thinking to myself that if you are well enough to speak to your lawyer on scene, there's no need for a paramedic. Of course, after expert advice from the unknown party on the phone, the patient will start complaining about severe neck or back pain and a headache to boot.

Each time, I have to take deep breath and remind myself that I was requested to respond and it is my job to be nonjudgmental and to legally protect myself by dotting my i's and crossing my t's. Don't get caught up in their nonsense—do the right things in the right way always!

51

Responding on September 11, 2001

It was a day that will live in infamy, a day that we will never and should never forget, a day when too many gave all. One thing is for sure, we all remember where we were and what we were doing, but none of us knew what was going to happen or how it would change our lives.

When you find yourself in a crisis situation similar to September 11, you will need to rely on your instincts from learned behavior. This is what happened on that day, but on a grand scale.

Immediately after the office of emergency management and the mayor's office realized the totality of the situation at hand, an all-call was made to both FDNY and NYPD. Following a strict emergency management plan and using their incident command systems, they set up a command center, and information started to flow.

As an individual, I knew my role, and it didn't include a fast track into the city. To be honest, that's all I wanted to do, but I knew that it was not the right thing to do. In moments such as these, discipline is of the essence and situational awareness is mandatory.

Not knowing what would happen or where I would be, I did what I was supposed to do. I came to my agency's headquarters and waited for our leaders to determine how we could be of assistance to the thousands we thought would be injured.

The moral of this story is that emotional maturity and discipline are needed to ensure we provide a balanced response to an emergency. Respect command and control, and understand the function of incident command.

52

Narcan, Anybody?

There is an equal and opposite reaction to every action you take, and this was precisely the case when they implemented ISTOP protocols, requiring all physicians to register opiates prescriptions online. The philosophy was to reduce the number of prescriptions written by different doctors at the same time.

The hypothesis proved itself; however, they had not thought of the unintended consequence of raising the street cost of prescription medications from one dollar per milligram to ten dollars per milligram.

In reality, the vacuum of prescription narcotics on the streets was quickly filled by slick heroin dealers looking to make a buck by selling heroin at three dollars a bag.

The difference between 20 mg of OxyContin and a bag of heroin is the precise dosing and absorption rate. Not to mention the fact that heroin dealers find it necessary to lace their product with fentanyl or some other potent synthetic opiates to boot.

It has caused a sheer pandemic, with over nine hundred deaths in New York City just in 2014–2015 alone. From big cities to small hamlets, everybody now knows someone who is using or has lost a loved one to an accidental overdose.

Lately, it seems to be a daily occurrence to administer Narcan or to find another lifeless body in a dark alley or a parent's basement.

In the case of heroin, one time might just be once too many!

53

Ambulance Driver

You know that show *Kids Say the Darndest Things*? It is awesome entertainment, and I often wonder where these kids get their information from. It's certainly a great laugh and very cute.

What is not so cute is what will happen if I get called "ambulance driver" one more time. I didn't go to college to study for hours and go to field training to complete many more hours of work to be referred to as an "ambulance driver." I have nothing against volunteers who drive ambulances and actually tip my hat to them for dedicating their time to volunteerism. What frustrates me is the general public's lack of understanding of the role a paramedic plays in today's health-care environment. We do so much more than just transport a patient safely from point A to the nearest appropriate hospital.

Is this total ignorance on the part of the public, or is it because of our failure to market our profession by telling the public about what we do, what we know, and how we save lives every day? Of course, it is the latter of the two scenarios.

So instead of getting angry and frustrated every time someone calls you an ambulance driver or EMT, take a few moments to educate the public with a short elevator speech you have prepared that describes what you do and how well you do it.

We ourselves are often to blame for the misunderstandings about our profession.

54

Practicing My IV Skills

One of the skills that set me apart as an EMT-Intermediate from being an EMT was starting IVs. I thought I was so cool and special. I'm sure you felt like that too when you started your first IV, or maybe you were shaking in your boots and too nervous to notice.

In the early '90s, while in class for my EMT-Intermediate and EMT-Critical Care, it was standard practice to start IVs on your classmates to gain competency. Actually, we had so much fun with it that we would challenge one another to get the largest bore needles into the smallest veins.

How we didn't end up with phlebitis or cellulitis is beyond me, but no harm was done other than having an arm full of puncture marks and the occasional black-and-blue mark.

Things have changed over time, and we no longer allow this practice in most programs due to liability. Damn lawyers ruin everything!

So how do you gain the experience necessary to get the most difficult sticks in the worst-case scenarios and environments?

You better get creative by stealing the neighborhood cat and start practicing. Just kidding, don't do that, of course—but you should find a piece of tubing and practice starting IVs with your right hand, left hand, on your side, and even upside down.

Worst-case scenario, you have your EZIO come to the rescue to provide your patients with the essential fluids or medication.

Practice makes near perfect.

55

Community Paramedicine

In this scenario, I'm referring to those of you who have grown up in the neighborhoods where you now serve as a paramedic.

I have lived and worked in the same township for the past twenty years. It's both a great honor and a tremendous stressor to take care of your own family, friends, and neighbors.

I'm fortunate to say that my roots only go back a few decades; however, I work with some medics who were born and raised right on this block.

Every time the tones go off, you never know whom you will be treating, knowing at times it will be someone you've known for a long time.

We have taken care of our teachers, police officers, firefighters, business executives, farmers, friends, and their kids, of course.

Although these calls are emotionally charged, as a *Positude* Paramedic, you set aside your emotions and get to work. It is only after the call that you can switch back to being a friend, family member, or neighbor.

You also need to recognize when it's time to step away and let your partner take charge, if that is possible.

The only advice I have for a paramedic working in his or her own community is to stay focused on the task at hand, treat each person like a VIP, and withhold your emotions until after the call ends.

56

What the Future Has in Store for Us

This is really a multitiered question and something all of us should consider. If I could see into the future, I would play the lottery and stretch out on a beach with a cold Mountain Dew and a good book in hand. Since I'm not a fortune-teller, let's get back to reality and take time to reflect on an excellent question.

Since we have no crystal ball, you are in charge of your future. You need to reflect on the information and data available and set realistic goals for yourself.

Here's a word of caution for each of you since I had to learn this the hard way myself. Being a paramedic is a heavy-lifting job and is taxing on your body. You need to not only take care of yourself now but also think about your future.

Do you have the right insurance? Is your body in the shape it needs to be to do this job?

Since we don't know what tomorrow brings, you need to be prepared for the worst-case scenario by maintaining a substantial bank of sick hours and developing alternate career options.

The future rarely delivers what we plan out so carefully. However, as *Positude* Paramedics, our glasses remain half-full, and we maintain a nimble mind-set that allows us to adjust on the fly.

An ounce of prevention is worth its weight in gold.

57

Participating in a Research Project

Do you want to be on the leading edge of science or be trailing along behind it? The only right answer for a *Positude* Paramedic is to be on the leading edge and to be part of the initial stages of innovation whenever possible.

Research can be broken down into two segments. You can participate in research projects to validate the efficacy of a new procedure, treatment, or medication. Or you can participate in research to develop new products, procedures, or medications.

Whenever the opportunity arises, you should take the opportunity to be part of either study. It will advance your status as an agency and a professional. Often, studies will come with funding to not only support the research project but also to provide the ability to engage and educate staff. If you take the opportunity and do well, you may have opportunities to travel and be part of development and beta testing.

If you play your cards right, you could get your agency's name and/or your name added to a published article. This could be a great boost for your agency to be recognized as being on the leading edge and for you to add professional enhancements to your résumé.

To get involved, all you need to do is a Google search with IHI, AHQR, JEMS, EMS Magazine, DOH, and the like.

Be part of the future, be on the leading edge of science, be an innovator, and be inspiring.

58

Joining the Mile-High Club

Get your mind out of the gutter already. Not everything is about getting lucky—or is it?

As you start your career in paramedicine, develop a strong future plan for yourself. Ensure it includes challenges that will push you to your natural limits, whether they're in flight, critical care, wilderness, or community medicine. Keep it exciting and something to look forward to. Whatever you choose for yourself, it should bring a level of professional satisfaction as well as fun.

I had the opportunity to join the mile-high club in 2003 when I joined *STAT* Flight Medivac Services out of Westchester Medical Center, Valhalla, New York.

It was at the top of my to-do list and my ultimate goal in my paramedic career. It is no secret that I love aviation and have held a private pilot certification for the past fifteen years, but it pales in comparison to flying a medivac helicopter.

If you have the physical stamina, aren't afraid of heights, and have a stomach that can withstand a bit of turbulence, I highly recommend that you too make it a career goal to join the mile-high club.

Providing critical medicine inside a sardine can with rotating wings is about the most exciting thing you will ever do in your life. If for nothing else, call your local medivac provider and request a ride-along to see what it is like.

Live without regret—fly high at every opportunity!

59

NYC Medics

By Sean Kivlehan

Swallowing deeply to suppress that nervous feeling you get when you encounter military personnel who speak a different language from you who are openly holding firearms in a foreign, nongovernment-controlled region, I asked what happened. It was around midnight, and I had been summoned to our "emergency" tent to evaluate a patient who had been injured in an accident. My experiences in New York City both as a paramedic and as an EMS educator had been both challenging and rewarding, but they could not have fully prepared me for providing postearthquake disaster relief in the North-West Frontier Province (NWFP) of Pakistan.

Just a few days earlier, I was working with a paramedic unit in Midtown Manhattan, preoccupied by an upcoming genetics test. (I was also a full-time undergraduate student at a school not far from my ambulance station.) Walking home from work, I received a phone call from another paramedic at my station, who asked, "Do you want to go to Pakistan?"

Sure, someday, I thought—but he had bigger plans. He was coordinating a group of responders to provide medical care to those in need following the 2005 Kashmir earthquake. It took some major schedule rearrangement, but within a few weeks I was on a flight to Islamabad. I was part of the second team deployed to the area, and by this time the group was formalizing into what is now the international disaster relief nongovernmental organization (NGO) called NYC Medics.

My perspective broadened quickly during my time in the NWFP after the earthquake. As part of a small group of paramedics and physicians, I provided medical disaster relief for survivors who'd had their villages crumble around them. More than any other experience, this changed me. Observing a way of life entirely different from mine forced me to reevaluate almost everything I took for granted. In New York, if you have a fever you can purchase some medicine at the local pharmacy or call 911 for an emergency. Things are different for the Pashtun of Garhi Habibullah, where medicine is often a myth and there is no emergency room.

Although the earthquake worsened already precarious living conditions, it also focused much-needed international aid and attention on a largely forgotten region. Simple preventative measures, such as telling people to avoid contaminated water or disseminating pamphlets on scabies, improved scores of Pashtun lives, as did routine medical procedures that so many Americans take for granted. The unending gratitude of a mother following the treatment of her child's diarrhea-induced dehydration solidified this feeling. She was so amazed to see a condition that many children do not survive so rapidly reversed.

We worked alongside Cubans and Iranians, which made me realize how easily the pursuit of a common goal can overcome cultural barriers. Differences soon became tools to help fill gaps, better preparing us to provide the best possible care to the greatest number of patients. Field hospital tents have little room for political or social boundaries: patients and their needs fill every square inch of space, and with each patient comes an invaluable opportunity to learn. In particular, I recall an elderly man who explained his religion and its traditions at length while his infected wounds were treated by antibiotics.

Once back home, it quickly became clear to me that working as a paramedic would no longer satisfy my craving to make a difference. I wanted to affect the change that was needed around the world, and to have any hope of that, I needed to better understand health care and public health as well as international politics. This drove me to attend medical school, complete a master of public health degree in international health, a residency in emergency medicine, and then a fellowship in international emergency medicine.

I deployed a second time with NYC Medics to Haiti in 2010 following the earthquake there, and they have grown into a much larger organization that deploys small teams of providers to emergencies around the world. My experiences with them pushed me to my current job in the Division of International Emergency Medicine and Humanitarian Programs at the Brigham and Women's Hospital and Harvard Medical School in Boston, where I work with many agencies to research and solve the problems facing people around the world who suffer from disasters and lack of access to emergency care, such as the victim of that car accident back in Pakistan.

60

Going from Medic to Medical School

I always wanted to play a doctor on the big screen. That's about as close I got to going to medical school. Actually, if this and that had not happened, my dream would have been to be a trauma surgeon or pathologist, but this and that *did* happen, which derailed my dreams for the time being.

I'm proud to say that I have worked with at least six partners who did stick to their dreams and today practice medicine in emergency rooms across the country. Each would tell you that they are a better MD/DO today because they were medics first. It allowed them to develop essential skills and practice strategies that allowed them to become highly effective medical investigators before ever touching a patient as a medical student.

As paramedics, we meet many people along the way who are curious about what we do. They ask pertinent questions, but none are better than those asked by youth corps members. These young people are aspiring doctors who join the local volunteer youth corps to become emergency medical technicians and gain valuable volunteer hours that will enhance their meager résumés in preparation to compete for a spot in their university of choice.

I have seen so many come full circle: all were EMTs and some become medics before going on to medical school. I'm like a proud parent, seeing those I coached and mentored graduate as medical doctors to pursue their dreams to deliver care to those in need.

By proxy, I'm part of their experiences and accomplishments, and that gives me great joy.

61

Giving Back

Go back over your own career or path to where you are today. How many people assisted you along the way? Think about your mom and dad, brothers and sisters, aunts and uncles, friends, colleagues, and bosses alike—each provided essential support to get you from point A to point B.

Now it is your turn to give back and keep the circle of giving intact.

I too had to learn the importance of giving back. It didn't come naturally until I reached a level of emotional maturity where I could see how others supported me.

Giving back doesn't have to be big. It just needs to be meaningful to the recipient. You can coach a local soccer team, be a den leader for scouts, or volunteer at the local soup kitchen.

Nothing is more powerful than mentoring a pupil who is still developing. As a paramedic, just look around you. We are surrounded by aspiring young doctors, nurses, and maybe other paramedics.

You can give back by sharing your experience by teaching, coaching, or mentoring on a variety of subjects.

Teaching is learning, giving back is sharing, and sharing is caring. It should be part of your everyday life.

I have the pleasure of mentoring four to five aspiring leaders at any given time. I learn as much from them as they do from me. They give me purpose, energy, and the inspiration to give back more.

Try it for yourself by making it a priority in life!

62

Paying It Forward

I'm not much of an Oprah fan, but I watched her shows on a regular basis while on duty with one of my female partners. She covers a different topic each day, but none of them were too memorable except for one.

Paying it forward is a powerful way to send a positive message to the receiver. It will often come as a total surprise, eliciting a genuine response of sheer joy and happiness. It will do the same for you if you have no expectation of anything in return. Bringing a smile to someone's face who doesn't expect it at all is one of the most powerful ways to show your deep care for humanity at large.

It doesn't take much to bring a smile to someone's face. Be creative in how you pay it forward. Think of little things that are low cost but have great impact.

Next time you are at the grocery store, assist a senior with pushing a cart or bring some goodies to the senior center.

Next time you are in line at the cafeteria, pay for the person right behind you. Don't say anything at all; just watch his face when he finds out that you paid the bill.

When you're asked what it is all about, simply ask that person to someday pay it forward for someone else.

Giving back or paying it forward is part of the typical actions of a *Positude* Paramedic. Make this part of who you are and what you do.

63

A Bad Boss

Bad bosses can be...yellers, screamers, blamers, or finger-pointers, and never at themselves, of course. How in the world do these people get into leadership positions? Liars, cheaters, manipulators, and con artists are just additional flavors of bad bosses.

Any or all of these kinds of bosses can be frustrating to work with or for. You will always be second-guessing their true motivation and know that they will not have your back in any situation.

Of course, not all bad bosses are badass; they come in all kinds, sorts, and flavors from a little bad to really bad. However, you will know one when you see one.

What are you supposed to do when you come across a bad boss, especially if you are still in the early years of your career? You have to learn to recognize a bad boss before you are on the receiving end of the abuse. Avoid making a commitment with the hope for change in attitude and behavior. A leopard doesn't change its spots.

If you found out about your boss only after you have been on the job for a while or if you happen to work for an episodically manic boss, you need to learn to avoid the highs and not be pulled into the lows. You will not be able to change the person—only your boss can do that for himself.

If you feel abused, document the events, seek advice from your peers, and if possible, go to HR to file a complaint.

Directive leadership should be a thing of the past; however, as long as staff members and the boss's boss are not willing to put an end to it, it will continue to exist. You don't need to be part of it!

64

Stress Debriefing

I'm tired, depleted, and emotional, and I feel like crying! This is what I felt like after so many separate incidents. Can you imagine a six-foot-five, 280-pound man crying like a little baby? It's not like it would be a bad thing to do so. Everybody is a little different in the way he or she deals with stress.

What I do know is that if you have a heart and soul, some 911 calls will draw out your emotions. I remember resuscitating a seven-year-old after he had been thrown from his car together with his twin brother. We fought hard and tried everything but to no avail. Thank God his brother made it, but it left all of us in an emotionally vulnerable state of mind. This could have been our son or brother—it truly hit home.

The question is, do we deal with this internally or seek professional assistance from a critical stress-debriefing team? Each of us will learn to deal with emotional trauma in his or her own way, but just don't deny your emotions as they will come back to bite you at some point in time.

Posttraumatic stress disorder is real, not just a perception. We are in a profession where we have chosen to run toward chaos and not in retreat. This comes with stresses unknown to many.

Don't wait until it is too late. Don't let your emotional immaturity stand in the way of getting professional help either individually or in a group. Talk about it a lot, go through the stages of grieving together with your team, and don't drown your sorrows in alcohol or drugs.

Stress is real, and it is part of our jobs. Be responsible and seek assistance when assistance is needed.

65

Doing the Right Things Right

What would happen if a Formula One driver cuts corners to get around the track? Does he significantly increase the chances of a spin out or even a crash? Absolutely, and when he wins, you could justify every corner he cut to get to the finish line first. However, if something goes wrong, the driver's life could be at stake, and most often the driver will retrospectively feel that cutting corners was not worth the risk.

In reality, we are often driving too fast, rushing our procedures and responses to the nearest appropriate facility. It is all well and good until it all goes wrong. If you are in doubt of this fact, Google "ambulance crashes," "HEMS crashes," or "EMS malpractice lawsuits."

Soon you will see that cutting corners is often a contributing factor to poor outcomes.

You have been taught to do the right things in your paramedics class, but you will find out that it is not necessarily the way it is done on the streets. What you need to be mindful of is the fine line between doing it easier or faster versus doing it the right way each and every time.

Doing the right things in the right way will lead to better outcomes with less variability. When lives are at stake during critical procedures such as intubation or EZIO insertion, you should use a checklist approach to ensure that the procedure is done correctly to optimize outcomes. Failure to do so will lead to leaky cuffs, intubating the esophagus, filling a third space with fluids, or, in the worst-case scenario, causing a life-threatening infection.

Plaintiff lawyers don't like it when you do the right things right!

66

Hospital Rotations

In 1993, I decided to study diabetic ketoacidosis as part of my final assignment. I took hours to research the topic and learn as much as I could. It was certainly interesting, but it was nothing like the real thing.

Theory can be kind of boring, especially when books are written for academia and not for adult learners who like to relate learning to real-life events to better lock in the information.

I don't remember precisely, but I think that the final report was about fifty pages. Although diabetic ketoacidosis is interesting to study and write about, you don't really realize its impact on a human body and its vital systems until you see a patient who comes into your emergency department with values at a critical level from their norm.

This was actually one of my patients on a rotation at a hospital upstate. This patient was in accurate distress, severely dehydrated, and in critical condition—everything I had studied right in front of my eyes.

I assisted ED personnel with resuscitation of this female patient by giving insulin, potassium, bicarb, and lots of fluids. The patient was intubated and placed on a ventilator. We thought we had turned the corner when her last blood gas came back more favorable. However, there was no change in Potassium.

After a short battle, the patient expired but not due to lack of trying to save her life. Bringing your books to life is still the best way to learn and retain.

67

Being a Great Mentee

Mentees literally come in all sizes, shapes, smells, and levels of intellect. If you do this long enough, you will meet one in each category. As a mentee, you have a responsibility to your mentor to conform, and this might take a critical feedback session to get a vital message across that will lead to change.

Since we all have been mentors at one time or another, we need to set clear expectations with our mentors right from day one.

As a mentee, your responsibility includes being on time, being prepared, and knowing what you want to get out of the shift, whether it is in the hospital, medic truck, medivac, or in the ambulance.

Preferably before you see your first patient, ensure that you have a common understanding and common knowledge with your mentor on expectations and abilities. Ask your mentor what a successful tour would look like. It will give you both the ability to strive for a common goal.

Ask lots of questions (but not too many) to show that you are interested in learning. Participate in the daily duties of checking equipment, checking expired medications, and cleaning and organizing as needed. Remain active by reading, studying, or watching educational videos. Only kick up your feet if your mentor says you can.

Being a mentee comes with lots of responsibilities; however, if you play your cards right, you will get the most out of these experiences, and this will translate into better knowledge, skills, and abilities.

68

Being an Even Better Mentor

Some of my finest memories are as a coach or mentor. It is truly a privilege to be trusted to teach someone with less knowledge. I have worked with mentees far smarter than I am and have learned as much from them as they did from me.

Being a mentor is being a leader. It is your responsibility as a leader to create an environment for learning, sharing, and relating.

There's no one way of mentoring since individuals are very different from one another. If you fail to identify how each of your mentees function, many of your instructions might fall on deaf ears.

As a mentor, make sure you take the time to get to know your mentees: discuss what is important to them and what they expect to get out of their time with you. In return, you will make adjustments to the way you mentor to meet the needs of each mentee. This will ensure an optimized and safe environment for all parties involved.

One of the most important things you can do is debrief your mentee at the end of your shift. It's a time for shared learning, discussion, and improvement.

As a mentor, live by the following rules to maximize success:

- Unwavering mutual respect
- Common knowledge
- Common understanding
- Being teachable

Teaching is learning; learn to teach.

69

Communicating without Talking

What is the likely reason why a process fails? It is most likely due to a failure to communicate. Why then am I bringing up the topic of communicating without talking?

At some point in time, you will be face-to-face with an emotionally disturbed person who is agitated and unstable in every sense of the word. It will only take a movement or a wrongly received word to set her off.

Another scenario to consider is a very loud and busy environment such as a car accident requiring extrication. You are in the backseat covered with sheets and trying to relay a message to your partner.

You get my drift—you can see yourself in many different scenarios where communication in the traditional sense is going to be senseless or at times even dangerous.

Communicating without talking is not something that you and your partner can develop on your first shift together. It takes time and dedication plus some trial and error to gain competency. Practice makes perfect.

I have worked out a system with my steady partners that allows us to communicate effectively and anticipate each other's next move without speaking more than necessary.

Your safety and that of your crew is at stake if you don't learn how to communicate with your body movements and predictable next options in a treatment plan such as suctioning, cricoid pressure, and so on.

Learn to read body language—both that of your partners and your patients.

70

Knowing Your Stuff

Remember that one person in your course who knows everything, has done every skill, and has seen all the gross injuries or experienced all the different illnesses? We all had that one person in our class.

You don't want that label of know-it-all, but you do want to feel confident that you know your stuff.

Knowing your stuff is exceptionally important, but it needs to be done with great humility. You owe it to your patients to keep learning at all times.

Carrying out your duties with great confidence and humility will provide a safe environment to learn, teach, mentor, and coach. Patients and crew members alike will feel comfortable around you as a care provider and be more receptive to your treatment modalities if you cultivate this safe environment.

The vital part of knowing your stuff means that you can identify and locate your equipment in pitch-black darkness or in the middle of a chaotic scene.

Keep asking great questions, and surround yourself with smarter, wiser, and more confident partners. Learn from the best and share with the next generation.

Submerge yourself in your profession to get the most out of it. Your patients will sense your confidence and notice your abilities in the way you treat them.

We can never know enough, so keep learning.

71

I Will Never Forget That "HOWL"

Sadly, I have been at too many accidents or joined police officers in too many notifications of such tragic events, but none stands out more than an accident in 1996.

It was a beautiful, sunny afternoon when we were dispatched to an MVA on a backcountry road. About five minutes into our response, we received an update from dispatch that prepared us for an ugly scene with critical injuries. This was not foreign to us, of course, but what we found was one of a kind.

A small car full of teenagers had literally wrapped itself around a telephone pole. I ended up extricating the front-seat passenger from the foot compartment—she was unresponsive and in critical condition but still alive.

We did everything we could—intubated her, decompressed her chest in four locations, and started a bilateral line of RL—without really making a difference. It was clear that she had suffered severe head and chest injuries.

Our hospital was not that far away, and the trauma team was ready to take over care. We collectively did everything possible for this beautiful thirteen-year-old girl to live but to no avail. This is the ugly part of our job, and we learn to deal with it.

What we were not prepared for was her father's reaction as he barged into the trauma bay unannounced and found his little girl naked on the table with too many tubes coming from everywhere. He jumped so high and screamed so loud that it has stuck with me forever. As a father of five, I hope that I will never be in his position. Hug your kids tight every day because you just never know.

72

Medic versus Doctor

I can tell you at least fifty of these stories, all with similar outcomes, but I will spare you the other forty-nine and tell you just one.

Too many years ago, we responded for a pedestrian struck on a busy highway. We had to travel at least ten minutes before we arrived on scene.

By that time, many bystanders had gathered, and usually in these types of cases, someone steps up to render first aid. Normally he or she would relinquish care the second we arrive on scene and feel relieved to step back.

This is true unless, of course, that person is a medical doctor who thinks that he is the patient's saving grace and that only he can provide definitive care in a prehospital setting. He will start barking orders like he is in his local emergency room. Now, if this was an experienced trauma surgeon or ED doctor, I would not mind the assistance and would even allow him to assist if we deemed him competent.

Of course, this doesn't ever happen; instead the doctor who is barking orders is an ENT, a podiatrist, or a cardiologist who has not seen any significant trauma since finishing up residency many years ago.

This patient happened to have bilateral near amputations with compound fractures to both lower extremities. This particular gastroenterologist had held her long bones in line but failed to control the bleeding, nearly causing this patient to lose her life.

Always be respectful but also be assertive in taking over care if the responding doctor doesn't possess the right skill set.

73

CMEs the Right Way

When was the last time you went to a continuing medical education (CME) hour and remember more than 10 percent of the information that was provided? It is likely you don't due to the fact that our adult brains don't retain much more than 10 percent of what we are told; nor do we use more than 10 percent of the technology available in any of our gadgets.

CMEs are done the right way when they are designed for the adult brain; however, we still don't see this often enough.

In actuality, this handbook is written with the adult brain and attention span in mind. Short, powerful chapters with most of the fluff removed allow you to retain only the fast facts. Each chapter was designed to grab your attention and leave you with a thought or idea for improvement, since it is likely that you will only remember that fact going forward.

Therefore, CMEs need to have a balanced approach between didactic theory-based presentation and hands-on examples that reinforce your teaching points.

A respiratory lecture on asthma, COPD, or CHF should include the application of CPEP, intubation, and medication management.

A cardiac lecture should include hands-on practice listening to heart sounds or interpreting 12-lead EKGs.

Don't wait for someone else to change the format—you need to lead the way. This includes considering reducing a CME event to only thirty minutes, which is far more manageable for the adult brain.

74

Embracing the Next Generation

These new kids coming into our industry are a bunch of nitwits: they do nothing and know even less. Why should I take time to teach them if they are not teachable?

Think back honestly to the days when you came out of school and hit the streets for the first time. Were you any smarter, wiser, or really even ready to function at a high level? Likely not, with the exception that my generation still showed up on time (around thirty minutes before your shift started).

As senior representatives of our industry, we are the custodians, teachers, coaches, and mentors responsible not only for ensuring that our profession remains relevant but for advancing it to the next level of performance.

We need to embrace our newbies and guide them through the rough waters in a safe environment. We need to provide support systems to ensure their success. We need to be open minded about new ways of doing things and not get stuck on past practices.

As you will see, communication and social interaction have shifted from telephone calls or friendly but intense chats about life to using smartphones and their million apps.

Try to understand how this generation grew up and how different it was from your experience. Embrace new technologies, but at the same time teach the next generation the value of the past.

It is our responsibility to share, teach, coach, and mentor our newbies into becoming the next generation of professionals.

75

Trauma Team

When you see a real trauma team at work, you will know it. It's like musical chairs with a set script that is executed flawlessly by a midsize team of professionals.

Over the many years I've been a paramedic, I have seen groups of people working a trauma case cause unnecessary delays, unintended errors, or even worse, mistakes.

On the days when I brought in Level I traumas and saw a good team at work, it was truly mesmerizing. There was a clear leader who stood back to keep an eye on the bigger picture while individual specialists checked out systems and reported back positive findings. There were technicians executing procedures with grace and ease. Most importantly, they all knew their role, what needed to be done, and in which sequence.

As a paramedic, you will be that trauma leader in the field supported by EMTs, paramedics, police officers, and fire department members. A trauma response should be practiced to identify each role that must be played; however, this is rarely the case due to its many complexities.

This makes your role as the trauma team leader in the field that much more important. Stand back far enough to see the entire picture; request feedback from responders working on your patient to develop a complete picture. Provide clear and concise directives that can be easily understood. Work with a sense of urgency with the common goal to get the patient to a trauma center within the golden hour.

Understand your role and execute it with precision while being nimble to changes in status.

76

Stroke: A Family Disease

Alan is truly one of the funniest guys I have ever met. Full of zest for life, his ear-to-ear grin told stories without him saying a word.

His son happened to be one of my best friends, and his family is full of great people who contribute to society on many levels without asking for anything in return. Nothing but the best—living life to the fullest for cheer, health, and prosperity—should have happened for all of them.

All of a sudden, the world changed for Alan, his wife Ruby, his son, daughter, and grandchildren, not to mention all the other folks that Alan interacted with every day of his life.

A minor weakness quickly developed into a massive stroke that essentially paralyzed part of his able body. The days of running after the grandkids or playing baseball the way he wanted were now mere wishes that were likely never to come true, at least not at the level he wanted.

Because of his character and loving support from many, Alan didn't lose his identity but just had to limit his physical function and the speed of all his favorite activities.

Strokes truly impact the entire family, and it really takes a village to get them on the path of recovery. I've worn purple every Thursday for the past ten years and tell Alan's story on a weekly basis to remind my patients who refuse to take good care of themselves how the impact of a stroke will affect not only them but their families as well.

Stroke prevention is truly the best medicine. As a paramedic, be proactive in your approach and in discussion with your noncompliant patients.

77

Checklist

As a pilot, I have one main objective: to equal my takeoffs and landings, preferably with my wheels down and wings up. To accomplish this consistently with the least amount of variability, pilots use checklists extensively. Partly because of checklists, catastrophic accidents are kept to a minimum.

In health care, some two hundred thousand or more patients die in hospitals due to human error. To reduce the incidence of catheter-associated infections, pressure ulcers, or falls, checklists are now used to prep, insert, and maintain central lines, PICC lines, and Foleys as well as to prevent falls. It has been shown that using checklists in each of these cases has made an impact on the number of unnecessary infections or even death. More importantly, during root-cause analysis, it is frequently noted that staff members failed to use checklists as part of their standard work, which could have been a contributing variable to a poor outcome.

In EMS, we don't use checklists, nor do we research prehospital-acquired skin infections, cellulitis, or other injuries from procedures that paramedics apply during the care of an emergency.

In New York State, we have to maintain a minimum equipment list for any emergency services vehicle. To maintain these requirements, we utilize a Part 800 checklist from the New York State Department of Health for basic life-support equipment; however, we don't use such a checklist for advanced life-support equipment.

Variation in a process causes potential liability. Checklists used properly control variation and will therefore provide a more predictable outcome.

Checklists do save lives!

78

Giving a Report to ED Personnel

Talking about variability in processes or standard work as discussed in the previous chapter on checklists, giving a report should be done in a standard approach. However, each region or even sometimes an individual hospital has different requirements.

In the mid-1990s, an upstate trauma center required a full report via UHF radio approximately ten minutes prior to arrival. If trauma activation is required, needless to say, the earliest possible notification is warranted.

Meanwhile, a local community hospital in a more urban setting required a minimalistic report with only pertinent positive findings and the required services upon arrival.

Is either one better than the other? It's all in the eye of the beholder, and that varies from shift to shift.

Personally, you should report pertinent positives in a thirty-second report via the medical control phone followed by a more detailed report upon arrival, preferably giving it only once to all the team members.

Your report should be concise, clear, professional, and spoken loud enough for all team members to hear at one time. You should stick to pertinent positive findings and provide ranges of pulse, blood pressure, pulse oximetry, and other readings plus the medication administered and the effect (if any).

Just like a great patient interview, giving an awesome report to your receiving hospital will elevate your professional standings and recognition. Work on this frequently until you get it right.

79

Legible PCRs

To some of you reading this, writing a prehospital care report (PCR) is a thing of the past, now that you use tablets. To make sure this has an impact on both the tablet user and those who still use paper, the moral of this short story is about professionalism and legal documentation.

We live in a litigious society where patients won't hesitate to place blame on the health-care provider and at times may file a lawsuit that could involve you as a piece of the puzzle.

As a hospital executive, I review notice of claim (NOC) reports too often. When something goes wrong, lawyers tend to sue everybody who touched the patient from the time 911 was activated through the discharge of the patient.

If you think that this only applies to major accidents, gross injuries, or catastrophic outcomes, you'll find out that this is a misconception.

Most NOC reports are about patients who slipped, tripped, and fell in a public area or drivers who were rear-ended and injured their neck or back.

These injuries often look benign at the scene, which could lead to you underdocumenting your findings or even failing to treat to the level that is expected from a paramedic under normal circumstances.

It is your electronic or written prehospital care report that will go to court initially for review and judgment. If you are not detailed and professional, or if it is illegible, you will end up in court testifying in front of a jury plus you will be cross examined, which can be a less-than-pleasant experience.

Documentation is an extremely important part of your job!

80

Being the Best I Can Be

Be all that you can be.
—US Army slogan

As a *Positude* Paramedic, you will be in charge of many critical calls over the span of your career. Each event is unique and requires your full attention at all times. You too have to leave all your effort on the table each and every time. Only you can make that evaluation postevent to see if you met this standard or not.

There's another angle to this story: you need to assess each day before you start your shift if you have the physical or mental capacity to give it your all. Although I have not studied this and therefore have no scientific evidence of such, I suspect that many medics come to work and perform at much lower than 100 percent.

Before you commit to your shift, consider yourself. It's no different than a pilot making a judgment about his or her capacity to fly—ask yourself if you are ready to leave it all on the table. Are you physically and mentally capable of providing high-quality, safe care for your patients?

As previously mentioned, most paramedics still work multiple jobs to make a living. Because of this, paramedics are at risk for mental breakdowns and physical fatigue. I can certainly relate to this after four back surgeries and two fusions of my c-spine and lumbar region.

Take care of yourself, exercise regularly, eat a balanced diet, limit alcohol consumption, and try to sleep six to eight hours per night. I'm saying this to myself as well, and someday I will get it right.

81

We All Have Bad Days

In twenty-eight years of emergency services, I have never had a bad day...said nobody ever! I have been cranky, sick, fatigued, and in pain; it's all part of doing a difficult job. I can think of only a few occasions that my day was so bad that I had to call it quits in the middle of my shift.

The key to your success as a *Positude* Paramedic is to realize the point when you are in a bad mood, not feeling 100 percent, in pain, or just not quite right but are still feeling well enough to give it your all when the time calls.

When you have a sucky day, communicate this to your partners and ask for their leniency before the shift starts. We all have days like this, and as great partners we step up our game to assist the other.

Great partners have each other's back at all times as long as it stays in balance. Even great partners get tired of carrying someone day in and day out.

Recognize when you go through a string of bad days that exceed the time of a normal viral infection—three to five days. You should seek professional assistance to overcome whatever ails you, whether it's depression, fatigue, or a nagging injury.

Don't let your reputation be tarnished by your inability to be a supportive, caring, and contributing partner in care.

Don't be in denial about burnout, depression, or circumstances in your private life that impede your professional life. There's help for you. Just pick up the phone and call your local employee assistance program.

Be mindful of your mindfulness!

82

Being There for Your Partners

Synergetic partnerships can bring so much professional satisfaction and so many personal gains to your career. I have been blessed to have worked with some of the best partners ever. I have been there for them and they have been there for me. It's not unlike a good marriage: through thick and thin, through health and illness, till we reach an age we can't do this job any longer, we'll take care of each other. I'm sure I will be friends with some of them for many years thereafter.

My longtime partner Bernadette had three beautiful kids while working full time. I remember her first pregnancy with Jack the best simply because it was her first experience as a mother and I got to spend time with him for the months after her return to work. We were lucky to live in the neighborhood we worked in, so it was not uncommon for us to stop by to say hello to the kids. On more than one occasion, I fell asleep in their La-Z-Boy chair with Jack on my chest. It gave me pure joy that I got to share with my partner and her family.

Other times you can't be there for your partners, but instead you have to be there for those left behind. Sadly, we have lost some good medics all too soon along the way, and some of these losses would have been preventable if we had only known.

I will forever remember Neil, John, Wes, Walter, and Nancy, just to name a few. Each had a heart of gold and was taken from us too soon. As a partner and a friend, I still wonder if I did enough to make them feel great about themselves and support them through their illnesses.

Be a great partner always!

83

Response Times

How long should it really take to get to the scene? That's an impossible question to answer, especially knowing that some regions of the United States are so vast that response times can easily exceed sixty minutes. However, how fast you get out of the door is something that you can fully control.

It is your primary responsibility and your duty as a *Positude* Paramedic to respond with urgency no matter what the dispatcher tells you initially. This doesn't mean that you need to be unsafe or even skip going to the bathroom for quick relief; it means that you should stop what you are doing and start moving in the direction of your vehicle.

In my early years, I drove Code 3 all of the time and often too fast or faster than necessary. It was not until they placed cameras in our vehicles that I reassessed my own behaviors. I have made adjustments in my driving style to ensure personal and public safety as we respond to emergencies.

In some areas of the country they have adopted a code system to indicate the level of urgency. An Alpha response would be different from a Delta response; however, it does take dispatchers with emergency medical dispatch training.

The right way to respond is to have a steady response with a sense of urgency, regardless of if you go Code 3 or not.

Safety should always be first, with a little urgency on the side!

84

Family Members

If you do this long enough in the community where you live, you will likely have to respond to a family member's emergency. Actually, this is more likely to happen when you are off duty and your family member calls upon you to determine if there's a need for an emergency response.

This can really leave you in the lurch or in a pickle (whichever you prefer). Liability never takes a backseat even when treating a family member. I have seen it happen several times, especially when catastrophic injuries happen while playing at a family member's house or yard.

As paramedics, we are often challenged to treat our patients the way we would treat our own mom or dad.

Now that you have a family member in front of you in some sort of distress, you have some choices to make. Do you take charge of the call, or do you look to your partner to step in and take over? Can you really be objective, and is your family member willing to tell you the truth? Every scenario will be a bit different and will call for great judgment on your part to make the right decision.

The only bad decision is the decision you don't make. Most often undertreating is worse than overtreating. Since such scenarios are often unpredictable, I would like to give you the following advice:

- Provide care and kindness just like you would for your mom or dad.
- Provide medical treatment like you are treating a skeptical lawyer who is known for securing large lawsuits over minor errors in treatment.

85

Drunk Drivers

Besides child abusers, sex offenders, and ignorant people, drunk drivers are lowest on my list of deplorable people (to use a reference from Hillary Rodham Clinton).

I have been sober for nearly twenty-seven years and can honestly look in the mirror and say that I have never been intoxicated while driving or operating any vehicle. Therefore, I don't sit in judgment of others while violating the rule myself.

Drunk-driving accidents are 100 percent avoidable at all times. There's absolutely no excuse for ever driving while intoxicated. You are essentially driving with a finger on the trigger of a loaded gun. You will get away with it 98 percent of the time, but in the 2 percent that you do not, you leave a trail of destruction behind that hurts many more people besides the obvious victims directly involved.

As a *Positude* Paramedic, you can't allow yourself to sit in judgment as a scene unfolds. It is your duty to render care regardless of the circumstances or causes. We are professionals at all times.

You can, however, be a strong advocate against drunk driving, driving under the influence, or driving while distracted. Speak up and lead by example, and never violate the rule yourself, no matter what.

We recently lost a beautiful girl, Larisa Karassik, due to a drunk-driving accident. Her innocence was taken from her due to sheer ignorance and stupidity. I have seen the devastation on her family and friends up close. It's horrifying.

In Larissa's name, "Friends don't let friends drive drunk."

86

Making a Difference

What is your true motivation for being a paramedic? Is it your ego, or is it your need to contribute and to make a difference? To be honest, you can't do this job very well if it is just ego driven. You will be an outcast among civil servants who have chosen a life of service, whether it's with the fire department, police department, or emergency medical services.

Making a difference is not just saving a life. Making a difference is doing the little things right every time.

Making a difference is going above and beyond by staying behind to prepare a meal for a diabetic patient who refuses to go to the hospital after an episode of hypoglycemia.

Making a difference is taking your time to present a patient who was recently pronounced dead by cleaning up the scene and staging the patient for family to see.

Making a difference is being prepared for the unknown, allowing you to work efficiently with your partners to save a life.

Making a difference is being a great partner, coach, or mentor to your teammates or spending time in the community to teach CPR.

As a *Positude* Paramedic, make it your life's mission to make a difference because it is the right thing to do.

Be the difference you want to see!

87

Balancing Stress, Sleep, and Nutrition

I'm writing this chapter to myself with the hope that you will read it too. It has been my lifelong struggle to keep my health in balance.

Let's see what I have done to myself: five kids, two full-time jobs, a beautiful wife, and a white house with a picket fence. I'm at least forty pounds overweight and for some reason can't sleep more than four hours per night. Strangely enough, I pass my annual physical with flying colors and only take something to maintain my blood pressure below 140/90.

You get the picture. I'm out of balance, but I think it works for me more often than not. This is really not about me: it is about my family, friends, partners, and patients alike. It is important to be constantly pursuing balance at all times.

You will have good days, great days, and some bad days, and it's important that you counteract the bad to find balance.

I maintain balance through meditation, spending time with my family, and trying to eat the right things more often than not.

If you feel lost, seek professional help such as a life coach, a nutritionist, or a personal trainer. Surround yourself with people who talk the talk and walk the walk.

Listen, look, and learn. Never give up on finding a healthy balance between stress, nutrition, and physical activity.

88

Getting a Promotion

You have worked hard for the past five years and are now in the running for a supervisor position. Depending on the circumstances, which will differ from person to person and location to location, what have you done to ready yourself for a promotion?

All too often, we find that highly talented and high-performing technicians are promoted into management positions but are given little or no training on management or leadership.

Your natural abilities and willingness to take on new adventures will take you only so far before you start faltering or failing to reach the next level of performance.

In actuality, this happens because of the senior leadership's failure to nurture the new managers, a mistake that can be very costly to all parties involved. This is referred to as the Peter Principle. Too many great technicians have tarnished their reputation due to lack of skill, knowledge, and ability in regard to managing and leadership.

I wrote a book titled *Positude Leadership: 4 Strategies, 5 Skills, and 100 Experiences to Becoming a Positude Leader.* You can find it on Amazon.com, and I highly recommend it if you are considering management, are up for promotion, or are in a management role but not advancing the way you had envisioned.

Make sure you are ready to be promoted and ready to articulate why you are the right person for the right job.

89

EMS Conferences: To Go or Not to Go

What is the real reason why people go to a conference? Is it just one big party with like-minded people, or is it an opportunity to gain vital information to better prepare you for the next call? Only you can answer that question, of course.

Part of being a great medic or a *Positude* Paramedic is making a promise to yourself to be on the cutting edge of medicine and not to fall behind. This means that you should participate in conversation, subscribe to trade magazines, and attend CME events.

Life is about having fun and hopefully doing things you have great passion for. Going to a conference could actually be the perfect combination of staying on the cutting edge of your profession and having fun at the same time.

Although national conferences are some of the best in the business, don't underestimate the power of a local event where networking with partners in care can truly elevate the performance of your team to another level.

I have only gone to a handful of conferences over the span of my career, but I have organized and attended countless numbers of CME events. I learned something from each of them, and at a very low cost, I must say.

The lesson for this short experience story is the fact that continuous learning is part of who you are. Don't become one of those old dinosaurs.

Be cutting-edge material!

90

Potty Time: To Go or Not to Go?

It was the toughest choice I ever had to make, and you would never guess what I had to choose between. I'm physically still in distress and not sure which choice was the best one, but it worked out in the end.

Tell me what you would have done!

I was solo on a dark, rainy, and windy night in suburban New York. We had been running all night from job to job. My partner was on his way to the hospital with a rule-out MI. I almost made it back to the station when the tones went off once again.

"M25, respond to Bethune Boulevard for an eighty-year-old female patient in severe respiratory distress." My interest spiked and my juices started flowing. At 2:00 a.m., it usually means an acute pulmonary edema or congestive heart failure patient. Minutes could mean everything, especially for our patient, since the fluid in her lungs would cause significant anxiety along with shortness of breath.

As soon as I started my response, I started feeling some cramping in my gut. The pain only worsened as I got closer to the scene. I could not stop my response, and at the same time I didn't think I could render care without pooping my pants.

Once inside, of course this patient was filled to the top as I was about to burst from the bottom. I made the difficult choice and applied high-flow oxygen, sat the patient upright in bed, and asked the officer to keep the patient alert.

I made it to the toilet where I found great relief, which allowed me to provide great relief to my patient after a few shitty minutes of delay.

91

Priceless Experiences

If you ever need a reason why this is one of the best jobs in the world, look no further than the next three scenarios.

It was a cold Sunday morning when we were asked to respond for a female in labor. Most often it just means that we end up reassuring the patient and transferring her to the hospital where she will deliver in a controlled environment some twelve to eighteen hours later.

But not today. The second we walked in we could feel that she was about to deliver. We jumped into action and within minutes a beautiful and healthy baby girl was born.

Later that day, we responded to an elderly man not feeling well. He had a urinary tract infection and needed a ride to the hospital. Since his blood pressure was a bit low, I joined him and gave him some fluids en route. He gave me more than I could ever ask for—a vibrant discussion about the early years of his life including the Great Depression and World War II.

To finish our shift, we were urgently called to the house of an unresponsive female patient who wasn't breathing. We found her in full cardiac arrest. Lying on the floor next to her was a crying two-year-old. Luckily, she was still in ventricular fibrillation, and after a few quick shocks, she had a spontaneous return of vital signs. By the time we got to the hospital, she was once again alert and oriented.

Each of these experiences was priceless, although they rarely happen on the same day. You will have the opportunity to do similar responses on a daily basis.

92

It's Your Patient's Emergency, Not Yours

I cracked a joke some time ago and told my patient he had a "mangina" for whining like a little girl. I am reminded of this on a regular basis, and I'm sure it will come up at my retirement dinner along with a few other "Walterisms."

How many times will you respond to jobs that seem like complete nonsense to you? Just another patient fishing for sympathy or trying to get out of work for the day at our expense.

These types of calls can become very trying over time, especially on very busy days when you didn't get a chance to drink your coffee or you skipped a meal.

In fact, it's one of the reasons I got myself into trouble and received a patient complaint for lack of empathy.

We can never make ourselves more important than the patient's emergency, no matter how difficult it may be.

It is our duty to respond regardless of the reason or its validity. We have to be mindful to not be prejudiced against frequent callers or abusers of the system. Don't let your guard down as you will be burned when you underdiagnose or completely miss an underlying medical emergency.

Be mindful of your mindfulness, especially of your ability to remain open minded and empathetic. Allow it to be their emergency and not yours.

Watch out for burnout syndrome—it starts in scenarios just like this.

93

Giving Reports: Is Anybody Listening?

Do you ever feel completely ignored by emergency-room staff when delivering a sick patient? I don't mind so much when it's just a BLS patient, but when we bring a critical-care patient, I'd like someone to pay attention.

Delivering excellence in patient care must be applied across the continuum of care from the time the patient calls 911 till he is stabilized in the appropriate emergency room or beyond.

When we discussed partnerships, your partnerships also need to be across the continuum, including your relationship with emergency-room personnel. Often, due to rotating shift work inside of hospitals, you will rarely see the same nurses and doctors each shift you work.

Conducting and participating in CME or mortality and morbidity rounds are great icebreakers for discussing process efficiencies and establishing a common bond or understanding.

Great systems will have a triage nurse ready to receive your report upon arrival, while in other systems you might have to wait a bit to give your report to either the nurse or the medical doctor.

It's a fact of life and difficult to mandate a better service; however, if you take the time to give a precise prehospital report on the medical control hotline, you should expect the right resources to be available upon arrival, especially respiratory care with a vent or a CPEP patient.

If you feel ignored, for the sake of great patient care, tell your supervisor so it can be addressed appropriately.

94

That's Not What My Patient Told Me

One of the most frustrating times in a paramedic's career is when a patient tells you one thing and then tells a totally different story when she speaks with the receiving physician.

We have all been there, and there's little you can do to prevent it. It gives you a great reason to always be skeptical and continue to ask questions throughout the call.

One of my primary-care physicians developed a communication system with his patients called ask-tell-ask. It is especially helpful when speaking with the elderly or patients whose primary language is not English.

Start by asking pertinent questions related to their past medical history, medication, or current complaint.

After carefully listening, tell the patient what you heard her say in detail without asking any additional questions at this time.

Now, ask the patient to repeat what you said. This should tease out any discrepancies, or it will generate additional questions for clarification.

Try it the next time you interview a patient—it really works. However, it will not eliminate the issues with those patients who only trust a doctor or those who do not have all their mental faculties in order.

Don't be defensive about these discrepancies; it truly happens to all of us. Your treatment should never solely depend on what your patients say—it must be connected to physical findings as well.

95

Cascading Stress Syndrome!

We live in a world full of stress. Stress can be found all around us. Stress can come from our children, from our spouses, and from our work.

Nothing is worse than the stress you receive from your boss because he is stressed by his bosses. This is called cascading stress syndrome.

The question really is, can we stop this phenomenon, or do we need to learn how to manage this phenomenon?

We need to learn to recognize this syndrome in its early stages and find ways to manage the impact of your boss's stress upon you and your staff members.

Once recognized, we need to take a step back and be empathetic to this real or perceived stress that causes this negative reaction.

We often want to come to the rescue by providing solutions, but instead we should take an approach of careful listening. We need to learn to understand the problem and its root cause to be proactive in avoiding such stress inducers.

This is not always possible. Therefore, at times we are better served by staying clear.

Most importantly, we need to recognize when we cause stress to our workforce due to stresses from above.

Use stress-debriefing techniques such as exercise or meditation to find balance once again. You can also offer assistance by taking on a specific task that could assist or alleviate a stress that is causing the cascading effect.

Sometimes we just need to stay clear, as this too will pass.

96

My Smallest Patient

One of the greatest privileges you have as a flight medic is taking care of the smallest infants. My smallest was a little fella at just 395 grams and at a gestational age of just twenty-four weeks.

Before you ever get this privilege, you have to go through extensive training and meet strict clinical competencies. I had the fortune to learn from some of the best NICU nurses and doctors at Westchester Medical Center located in Valhalla, New York.

When we say a child is not a small adult, the same can be said that a full-aged gestational infant is not the same as a twenty-four-weeker whose eyes are still fused shut.

We got the call on an early morning to transfer a twenty-four-week-old gestational male neonate to our Level IV NICU.

Normally, our flight nurse will take charge of such calls, as the flight medic is responsible for all the procedures, transfer, and ventilator. I'm not sure whose job is more stressful. As great partners, we work off each other's strengths and weaknesses. We often worked in synchrony, which enhanced our abilities to provide excellence in care.

That morning like many before, we needed to overcome challenges with ventilation as the neonate's premature lungs clearly weren't ready to work as hard as they needed to. After some nerve-racking moments establishing an umbilical central line and finding the right pressure settings, we got on our way and delivered him without further incidence.

It truly is an honor to have taken care of these little peanuts.

97

Maintaining Competency

I'm going to administer eighty milligrams of Lasix for an obvious patient in congestive heart failure.

"Not so quickly," says my partner of many years. "Lasix is no longer a standing order and requires you to call medical control. Do you need some nitroglycerin spray instead?"

This is an example of staying on top of the latest medical control advisory committee guidelines based on established best practices.

This is not as easy as you might think it would be. I have administered lidocaine to at least five hundred patients with great results and few negative side effects. Suddenly, the orders were changed on weak research (in my opinion), and then we needed to administer amiodarone before lidocaine.

Good luck remembering that one in a crisis situation after your brain has been hardwired to go with lidocaine, which, by the way, comes in a prefilled syringe unlike amiodarone.

Medicine should not be about what I want it to be based on personal experiences. Medicine should be based on solid research and best practices. Money should not be a driver in this equation.

As a *Positude* Paramedic, it is your responsibility to maintain constant vigilance for better ways of doing something and to adjust your personal practice if a best practice has been proven to be more effective.

Stay up on your skills, knowledge, and abilities.

98

Applying a Tourniquet around Your Partner's Neck

This is only recommended if you untie every five minutes for thirty seconds. We all have had partners who were less than desirable, a situation that is especially tenuous when you are stuck with them for twelve to twenty-four hours. Playing hide-and-go-seek is in order to prevent World War III from breaking out.

Over the last quarter century, I have had about two hundred different partners with whom I worked for at least one shift. I am glad I can only recall a small handful who qualified for the tourniquet treatment.

Some were outright liars and thieves or were deplorable, unsanitary, or plain dangerous as medics. At times, these undesirable traits were accentuated due to conflicting personalities. By the grace of God, nobody ever got hurt or killed along the way.

Most of the paramedics I know can be identified as alpha personalities. They are the key drivers to our best practices and desirable clinical outcomes...until you put two alpha personalities together when neither can adjust to take second seat. This is a recipe for disaster.

Therefore, it is your responsibility to know when to lead and when to follow. It all starts with effective communication between partners or teams.

If you find you are in conflict with a partner who is not open to dialogue or critical feedback, seek advice from your supervisor. If you find out that your partner is doing something unethical, report him or her immediately.

When in doubt, apply tourniquet and notify your boss!

99

Never Too Much Coffee

The finer moments in life: a good cup of coffee from Starbucks, Dunkin' Donuts, or 7-Eleven. It's the right way to start your day.

There are couple things you need to remember about drinking a fine latte, a Frappuccino, or just a cup of plain dark roast.

Coffee (or *Koffie* in Dutch) is a potent diuretic that will make you want to go pee at the least opportune time. Drink with caution.

Coffee or a cappuccino is not a wake-up kind of a drink. To get the greatest effect from your coffee, you should drink it before you lie down for a nap. By the time you wake, the caffeine is at its optimum point, giving you its maximum effect to be alert and oriented once again.

Do you know people who say that they can't drink regular coffee late at night because it prevents them from falling asleep? Studies have actually shown that you can fall asleep but not *stay* asleep. If you are one of those people who need eight hours of sleep per night, don't drink coffee late at night and you will feel better in the morning.

Coffee is like a fine wine: the beans need to be roasted just right to enrich the flavors to make it an oral delight.

You can never have too much coffee—morning, noon, or night. Try different coffees from around the world, and you'll be surprised what can be done with a little green bean.

100

I LOVE MY JOB!

Passion, skills, knowledge, and ability are the four key qualities you should possess when functioning in a job you love.

I know lots of highly skilled and knowledgeable paramedics who lack passion and/or abilities. All of them are miserable in what they do. Their partners and patients often suffer the consequences from their low behavioral capacity or emotional maturity.

I'm truly the luckiest guy on this planet. I still feel passionate about what I do and about the difference I want to make.

Because of some highly talented instructors, teachers, and partners, I gained the skills necessary to do this job well.

I never stopped learning, exploring, and staying on the leading edge of paramedicine, which has allowed me to be knowledgeable about my trade to the first degree.

I have been fortunate to have been selected and entrusted to provide services as a paramedic, critical-care paramedic, and flight paramedic. In these roles, I gained the ability to execute my knowledge and skills day or night, rain or shine, hot or cold.

I love being a *Positude* Paramedic and hope that you will be as lucky as I have been for many years.

Being a paramedic is the best job ever, bar none!

Conclusion

A couple hundred pages and some fifty thousand words later, I truly hope that you, as an aspiring paramedic, have found the right reason to pursue this awesome job.

For our new paramedics just out of school, I hope you have learned from my experiences and will avoid some of the same pitfalls and strengthen your identified weaknesses. You are starting your journey to becoming a *Positude* Paramedic or are on your way to medical school or beyond. Never forget those who came before you or where you came from.

For the more experienced paramedics among you, I hope that you were able to relate to my stories and feel inspired to become a *Positude* Paramedic.

Throughout the text, I encouraged all readers to continue to learn, share, teach, coach, and mentor; it is your responsibility to elevate our profession to the next level of recognition and performance.

There are exciting times ahead of us, with lots of opportunities to shape new career paths for paramedics and to make our profession that much more relevant.

Get involved in your local high schools, colleges, and fire training centers to promote and encourage the next generation of *Positude* Paramedics.

Relate; don't compare. And allow yourself to get to the next level of performance.

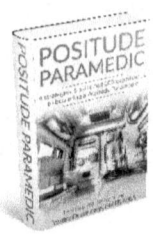

About the Author

Walter Dusseldorp, MBA, FACHE, EMT-Paramedic, has served the Hudson Valley for the past twenty-seven years in his capacity as a paramedic, lieutenant paramedic, flight medic, and president of the Hudson Valley Paramedic Association. He has focused his passion and energies on furthering the paramedic profession. Walter is seen by his peers as a *Positude* Paramedic and as a coach and mentor to aspiring students, volunteers, and paramedics alike. Walter wrote *Positude Paramedic* as a guide to making the *right* career decisions, asking the *right* questions, and developing evidence-based action plans. Walter also shares his personal experiences so that readers can learn by relating and not comparing.

Positude Paramedic is an outstanding handbook for paramedics in every stage of development. Written by paramedics for paramedics, the book's power comes from its short chapters and stories. It's a handbook that adds value and is designed with the adult learner in mind.

Special contributions include chapters by Jeff Rabrich, DO; Sean Kivlehan, MD; paramedics Lieutenant Bernadette Frae, Frank DiGianni, Joel Hirshfield Esq., and Lieutenant Steven Kanarian; and the Karassik family.

Positude Paramedic

4 Strategies, 5 Skills, and 100 Experiences to Becoming a Positude Paramedic

Walter Dusseldorp, MBA, FACHE

Being a *Positude* Paramedic literally means leading with a positive attitude.

How is this strategy different from all the others? Simplicity in its meaning and implementation—simply be *awesome* every day!

This strategy is not only intended for paramedics. I wrote the book from my perspective as a paramedic and referenced a variety of service providers throughout; however, our strategies and skills are highly transferable to any student who is searching for the right career path.

Being a paramedic who works with great passion, skill, knowledge, ability, and *positude* will most definitely enhance your likelihood of awesome clinical outcomes.

I challenge you as the reader to become a *positude* leader among emergency services, whether as a paramedic, police officer, or firefighter.

Feel inspired—be inspiring!

www.ingramcontent.com/pod-product-compliance
Lightning Source LLC
Chambersburg PA
CBHW071419180526
45170CB00001B/146